Jekabs Krastins

AKI- an underestimated problem in the pediatric intensive care

AF138168

Jekabs Krastins

AKI- an underestimated problem in the pediatric intensive care

LAP LAMBERT Academic Publishing

Impressum / Imprint

Bibliografische Information der Deutschen Nationalbibliothek: Die Deutsche Nationalbibliothek verzeichnet diese Publikation in der Deutschen Nationalbibliografie; detaillierte bibliografische Daten sind im Internet über http://dnb.d-nb.de abrufbar.
Alle in diesem Buch genannten Marken und Produktnamen unterliegen warenzeichen-, marken- oder patentrechtlichem Schutz bzw. sind Warenzeichen oder eingetragene Warenzeichen der jeweiligen Inhaber. Die Wiedergabe von Marken, Produktnamen, Gebrauchsnamen, Handelsnamen, Warenbezeichnungen u.s.w. in diesem Werk berechtigt auch ohne besondere Kennzeichnung nicht zu der Annahme, dass solche Namen im Sinne der Warenzeichen- und Markenschutzgesetzgebung als frei zu betrachten wären und daher von jedermann benutzt werden dürften.

Bibliographic information published by the Deutsche Nationalbibliothek: The Deutsche Nationalbibliothek lists this publication in the Deutsche Nationalbibliografie; detailed bibliographic data are available in the Internet at http://dnb.d-nb.de.
Any brand names and product names mentioned in this book are subject to trademark, brand or patent protection and are trademarks or registered trademarks of their respective holders. The use of brand names, product names, common names, trade names, product descriptions etc. even without a particular marking in this work is in no way to be construed to mean that such names may be regarded as unrestricted in respect of trademark and brand protection legislation and could thus be used by anyone.

Coverbild / Cover image: www.ingimage.com

Verlag / Publisher:
LAP LAMBERT Academic Publishing
ist ein Imprint der / is a trademark of
OmniScriptum GmbH & Co. KG
Heinrich-Böcking-Str. 6-8, 66121 Saarbrücken, Deutschland / Germany
Email: info@lap-publishing.com

Herstellung: siehe letzte Seite /
Printed at: see last page
ISBN: 978-3-659-68850-8

Copyright © 2015 OmniScriptum GmbH & Co. KG
Alle Rechte vorbehalten. / All rights reserved. Saarbrücken 2015

TABLE OF CONTENTS

1.Role of renal dysfunction in the pediatric critical illness

Acute kidney injury (AKI) is increasingly recognized as a cause of increased morbidity in critically ill children and adults, and damage to the kidney, a central mediator of homeostasis in the body, affects patient survival [Andreoli, 2002; Hui-Stikle et al., 2005]. AKI is now known to be an independent risk factor for mortality. The list of causes of AKI in pediatrics is long [Andreoli, 2009]; however, the true etiology is likely multifactorial, related to a combination of several factors, such as ischemia and reperfusion injury, disruption of renal vasomotor homeostasis, hypoxic and oxidative stress, and cytokine-driven effects. The kidney is central to numerous homeostatic control mechanisms, including water balance, electrolyte handling, erythropoiesis, vascular tone, acid–base status, and regulation of normal glucose metabolism. The laboratory indicator, glomerular filtration rate (GFR), is the accepted reflection of nephron function. Calculations of GFR rely on serum creatinine (SCr) and are often unreliable because of variability within age groups, gender, metabolic state, body composition, and excretion by the kidney itself [Schwartz et al., 2009]. Children usually do not have the comorbidities like diabetes, obesity, hypertension, cardiovascular disease, typical for adult patients. However, the epidemiology of AKI in children has changed over the past decade, from primary kidney disease, such as HUS (hemolytic uremic syndrome), to diseases in which the kidneys are affected as a result of another systemic disease or its treatment [Vlasselaers et al., 2009]. Critically ill children with multiorgan dysfunction or exposed to nephrotoxic medications represent the most prevalent pediatric cohorts who develop AKI [Hui-Stickle et al., 2005].The rates of AKI development in pediatric ICUs depend upon the populations studied and the AKI definition used, ranging from 4.5% (all admitted patients with AKI defined as a doubling of SCr [Bailey et al., 2007] to 82% (only children receiving invasive mechanical ventilation and receiving one or more vasoactive medications, with AKI defined by a 25% decrease in estimated SCr). Mortality is higher for children with AKI, especially those with multiorgan failure [Gallego et al., 2001]. Therefore all children with any of these risks factors should be monitored closely for the development of AKI. Early AKI detection is crucial, as even small increases in SCr may be associated with pediatric patient morbidity and mortality [Price et al., 2009]. Definitions of oliguria, the bedside indicator for AKI diagnosis, also are varied. Although clinicians have shown that sick kidneys affect morbidity independently and synergistically with multi-organ disease, study of the impact of kidney injury is limited by having to use these markers of failure. This review is focused on evidence-based AKI research, highlighting disturbing epidemiologic trends for pediatric AKI, novel detection strategies, the role of AKI as an independent causative agent of injury, and available evidence-based data regarding management and outcomes.

2.Etiology of AKI.

Traditional AKI causes are stratified into location of injury relative to the kidney. The diseases that fit into "pre-renal" and "intrinsic renal" share the commonality that they alter the regional perfusion of, and subsequent oxygen delivery to, the kidney. "Post-renal" injury refers to antegrade urine flow disruption from the kidney. The pathophysiology of AKI in the intensive care unit, however, is much more complex and multifactorial.

2.1.Altered Renal Perfusion.

The kidneys receive a high percentage (20% to 25%) of the cardiac output at any moment. Aberrations in the intricate regulatory mechanism in place to maintain renal perfusion pressure lead to injury such as acute tubular necrosis [Just, 2007]. Pediatric kidney transplant recipients of organs with increased ischemic times during harvest have increased rates of acute tubular necrosis [El-Husseini et al., 2005], as do patients with long cross clamp times during cardiopulmonary bypass (CPB) [Boldt et al., 2003]. Direct effects on renal blood flow in the microvasculature of the vasa recta occur in sickle cell disease, rhabdomyolysis, HUS, and tumor lysis syndrome.

2.2.Vasomotor Nephropathy.

AKI occurs by stress-mediated glomerular endothelial release of vasoactive substances, proteases, reactive oxygen species, and nitric oxide. For example, the factor XII plasma contact system, coagulation cascades, and complement pathways are activated in renal endothelium during CPB [Moat et al.,1993].

2.3.Sepsis and AKI.

Sepsis causes AKI in up to 50% of cases [Warady, Bunchman, 2000]. Although the precise mechanism remains unclear, a wide spectrum of cytokinesis implicated, as are circulating lymphocytes, T cells, and native kidney tubular epithelial and endothelial cells. Interestingly, septic AKI does not appear to be ischemia-dependent, because it can occur in hyperdynamic renal blood flow [Bellomo, 2008].

2.4.Aberrant oxygen homeostasis.

A natural degradation in oxygen tension exists from the level of the renal artery to the counter-current mechanism in the vasa recta, making the kidney highly susceptible to both hypoxic and oxidative injury during ischemia-reperfusion. Experimental ischemia leads to renal dysoxia, a situation also seen in sepsis, in which renal cells are unable to utilize oxygen for energy, regardless of oxygen availability [Legrand et al., 2008].

4

2.5.Nephrotoxins and AKI.

Nephrotoxic medications in the intensive care unit contribute to nearly 25% of AKI cases. Common offenders include aminoglycoside antibiotics, nonsteroid alantiinflammatory agents, radiopaque contrast, and immunosuppressives such as calcineurin inhibitors [Jones, Lee; 2008].

2.6.Associated syndromes.

AKI is seen in conjunction with pulmonary, hepatic, and cardiac failure [Price et.al., 2008]. The increased mortality reported with these dual-axis syndromes underscores the kidney's centrality to host survival. Although exact mechanisms are unknown, they all are almost certainly linked to aberrations in blood flow distribution and to endothelial activation [Moore et al., 2004].

3.Epidemiology of AKI.

One of the fundamental problems in interpreting studies in AKI has been the lack of a unified definition. There were discrepancies between the two more commonly used definitions, [Bellomo et al., 2004] leading to differences in incidence and outcomes of AKI. It was therefore essential to have an agreed definition for epidemiological studies, assessment of risk factors for AKI, evaluation of biomarkers predicting severity and recovery from AKI, and interventional trials. Pediatric AKI epidemiological study has intensified over recent years, likely as a result of more widespread provision of acute RRT modalities to critically ill children [Warady et al., 2004]. AKI rates appear to have increased by over ninefold from the 1980s through 2004 due to increasing use of more invasive management and higher illness severity of critically ill children [Vachvanichsanong et al., 2006]. Single center studies from the 1980s and 1990s report HUS, other primary renal causes, sepsis, and burns as the most prevalent causes leading to AKI [Andreoli, 2002]. More recent data [Williams et al., 2002] reveal a dramatic shift in the epidemiology of AKI, with the most common causes being renal ischemia, nephrotoxin use, and sepsis. Thus, in the current era, AKI more often develops in hospitalized children as a result of a systemic illness or its treatment and not from primary kidney disease, which is similar to the situation in adults. Another limitation of the past AKI studies was the lack of standardized definition. The incidence of the most severe forms of AKI, defined by dialysis requirement, ranges from 1 to 2% of all critically ill children [Bailey et al., 2007]. In children undergoing CPB surgery, the incidence of AKI is in the range of 10–50%, depending on the definition used [Boldt et al., 2003]. Even small increases in SCr, much less than would be considered indicative of the need for RRT, are now recognized to contribute to poor outcomes. Chertow and colleagues demonstrated that increases in SCr for 0,3 mg/dl were associated with increased adult patient mortality, even when outcome was controlled for significant patient co-morbidity [Chertow et al., 2005]. Similar results were noted in pediatric patients with acute decompensated heart failure; patients with a >0,3 mg/dl rise in SCr demonstrated a sevenfold increased mortality risk [Price et al., 2008]. These studies highlight the need for more refined AKI definitions for both children and adults and for a focus on earlier detection of AKI before a patient requires RRT.

6

4.Definition and classification of AKI.

Historically, a substantial rise in SCr and a drop in urine output have been used to determine if a child has AKI. Prior to the 2004, over 30 definitions of AKI existed in the literature which made comparison between studies very difficult. In 2004, the ADKI group proposed the RIFLE (Risk, Injury, Failure, Loss and End-Stage) classification definition of AKI [Bellomo et al., 2004], (Table 1).

Table 1. **RIFLE CLASSIFICATION AND STAGING SYSTEM[1]**

Stage	Serum creatinine criteria	Urine output criteria
Risk	Serum creatinine increase 1,5- fold OR GFR decrease >25% from baseline	<0,5 ml/kg/h for 6 hours
Injury	Serum creatinine increase 2- fold OR GFR decrease >50% from baseline	<0,5 ml/kg/h for 12 hours
Failure	Serum creatinine increase 3- fold OR GFR decrease >75% from baseline or serum creatinine $\geq$354 μmol/l (4 mg/dl) with an acute increase of at least 44 μmol/l (0,5 mg/dl)	Anuria for 12 hours

The first 3 categories (Risk, Injury and Failure) staged the degree of AKI based on whether the amplitude of SCr rise (or decrease in estimated glomerular filtration rate, eGFR) and/or a drop in urine output. The last two categories (Loss and End-stage) defined temporary or permanent loss of kidney function after AKI. In 2007, a similar definition (pRIFLE), (Table 2) was proposed for pediatric patients and has been used to describe several cohorts [Akcan-Arikan et al., 2007; Zappitelli, 2008].

Table 2. **pRIFLE CLASSIFICATION AND STAGING SYSTEM[2]**

Stage	Serum creatinine criteria	Urine output criteria
Risk	eClCr decrease by 25%	<0,5 ml/kg/h for 8 hours
Injury	eClCr decrease by 50%	<0,5 ml/kg/h for 16 hours
Failure	eClCr decrease by 75% OR eClCr<35 ml/min. per 1.73 m^2	<0,3 ml/kg/h for 24 hours OR anuric for 12 hours

Abbreviations: eClCr –estimated creatinine clearance

---

[1] Bellomo, R. et al., 2004
[2] Akcan-Arikan et al., 2007

The RIFLE definition was updated in 2007 by the Acute Kidney Injury Network [Mehta et al., 2007], by many of the same experts who proposed RIFLE. The AKIN definition) is similar to the first 3 stages of the RIFLE classification with a couple of changes. (Table 3).

Table 3.   **AKIN CLASSIFICATION AND STAGING SYSTEM**[3]

Stage	Serum creatinine criteria	Urine output criteria
1	Serum creatinine increase ≥23,5 µmol/l (≥0,3 mg/dl) OR increse to 1,5 to 2-fold from baseline	<0,5 ml/kg/h for 6 hours
2	Serum creatinine increase 2-3 –fold from baseline	<0,5 ml/kg/h for 12 hours
3	Serum creatinine increase >3 –fold from baseline or serum creatinine ≥354 µmol/l (4 mg/dl) with an acute increase of at least 44 µmol/l (0,5 mg/dl) OR need for RRT	<0,3 ml/kg/h for 24 hours OR anuria for 12 hours or need for RRT

Abbreviations: AKI, acute kidney injury; AKIN, AKI Network; GFR, glomerular filtration rate; RIFLE, Risk, Injury Failure, RRT, renal replacement therapy.

Recently, the Kidney Disease Improving Global Outcomes (KDIGO) [www.kdigo.org] has brought together international experts from many different specialties to produce a definition and staging system which will harmonize these recent definitions (Table 4). This classification and staging system now is validated also in the pediatric population [Selewski et al., 2014]. The first study which defined AKI using the pRIFLE criteria found that AKI occurred in 82% of critically ill children admitted to a ICU who received invasive mechanical ventilation and at least one vasoactive medication [Akcan-Arikan et al., 2007]. That is opposite to 4,5% prevalence of AKI in all patients admitted to the PICU [Bailey et al., 2007]. Worsening AKI defined by the pRIFLE criteria was an independent risk factor for mortality and increased hospital length of stay.

---

[3] Ricci, Z. et al., 2011

Table 4.   **KDIGO CLASSIFICATION AND STAGING SYSTEM**[4]

Stage	Serum creatinine criteria	Urine output criteria
1	1,5–1,9 times baseline OR ≥0.3 mg/dl (≥26.5 μmol/l) increase	<0.5 ml/kg/h for 6–12 hours
2	2-2,9 times baseline	<0.5 ml/kg/h for ≥12 hours
3	3 times baseline OR increase in serum creatinine ≥354 μmol/l (4 mg/dl) with an acute increase of at least 44 μmol/l (0,5 mg/dl) OR Initiation of renal replacement therapy OR, in patients <18 years, decrease in eGFR to <35ml/min per 1.73 m^2	<0,3 ml/kg/h for ≥24 hours OR anuria for ≥12 hours

Abbreviations:, eClCr –estimated creatinine clearance

The critically ill patient receiving invasive mechanical ventilation and vasoactive medications should prompt early vigilance for AKI occurrence. A recent publication proposed the concept of a "renal angina" to prompt investigation into the presence and causes of AKI, much as chest pain and associated signs and symptoms evaluation for acute coronary syndrome and myocardial infarction [Goldstein, Chawla, 2010]. The goal was to develop a simple score (RAI, renal angina index), which is easy calculable and can be used at the bedside [Basu et al., 2014]. Termed "renal angina", a three-tiered schema empirically places children into moderate (any ICU admission plus doubling of serum creatinine or fluid overload >15%), high (heart failure or stem cell transplant plus serum creatinine increase ≥0.3 mg/dl or fluid overload >10%), and very high risk for AKI (mechanical ventilation and vasoactive medication plus any increase in serum creatinine or fluid overload >5%). RAI is calculated by multiplying risk level (score 1-3) by injury level (score 1-8). Final result of RAI is expressed in numbers and varies from 1 (minimum risk) to 40 (maximum risk). Thus, as the AKI risk increases (e.g. mechanical ventilation), less evidence of AKI is needed (e.g. small changes in serum creatinine) to meet the threshold for renal angina. In analogy with cardiac angina, the major goal of renal angina determination is to identify children who will maximally benefit from biomarker measurement for prediction and early treatment of AKI. Now RAI is validated in multiple studies (Basu et al. 2014).

---

[4] Kidney International Suppl. (2012) 2, 19

5.Diagnostic Tools.

5.1.**Renal NIRS**. Near-infrared spectroscopy (NIRS) is a non-invasive, continuous method of evaluating real-time regional oximetry (rSO_2). The technology is based on the different absorption of near-infrared wavelengths by oxygenated and deoxygenated haemoglobin. The transmitter and the receiving optodes are placed ipsilateral in the sensor. Several studies have shown a moderate correlation between cerebral and somatic NIRS monitoring and markers of cardiac output such as lactate or systemic venous oxygen saturation ($ScvO_2$) and regional tissue perfusion in a variety of clinical settings [Hoffmann et al. 2004]. However, NIRS measurements in different organs have shown variable correlations to systemic oxygenation parameters or no reliable correlation at all. Minute to minute variations in somatic NIRS numbers may be correlative with low perfusion states, including hypovolemic pediatric emergency room patients [Hanson et al., 2009].

5.2.**Urinary pO_2.** Adult urine pO_2 levels, assumed to mirror changes in renal oxygenation, have been correlated to AKI [Kainuma et al., 1996].

5.3.**Magnetic resonance imaging**. BOLD (blood oxygen level dependent) magnetic resonance imaging have been used in adults to determine changes in renal parenchymal oxygenation [Han et al., 2008]. BOLD uses deoxyhemoglobin as an endogenous contrast agent to identify areas of reduced oxygen tension within the kidneys – resulting in decreased intensity on T2-weighted MR images. Although the various MRI-based techniques offer promise in our ability to investigate changes in renal perfusion in critically ill patients, it is difficult to imagine how they could be widely applied at this stage. The MRI environment is hostile to the critically ill and carries some significant safety concerns during transport and during a prolonged period in the magnet. In addition, obtaining high quality MRI scans in the critically ill is also often very challenging. The high cost adds a further degree of difficulty, which makes repeated assessment logistically very difficult.

5.4.**Ultrasonography.** Ultrasonography is the most commonly used imaging modality in the initial evaluation of patients with acute or chronic kidney diseases. It is widely available, easy to use, free of complication and can be performed at the bedside. Standard ultrasound provides information on kidney size (a small kidney suggests possible atrophy in the context of chronic kidney disease, a large kidney might suggest the presence of infiltrative disease), cortical thickness and echogenicity and enables imaging of the excretory tract to diagnose outflow obstruction. In AKI, however, standard ultrasound

11

examination is normal most of the time. Assessment of renal perfusion by ultrasound can be approached by Doppler techniques or with microbubble-based contrast agents (contrast-enhanced ultrasound). Blood flow quantification using contrast-enhanced ultrasound was first described by Wei et al. in a canine model [Wei et al., 1998]. Although in its early stages of validation, contrast enhanced ultrasound seems to be a promising technique to evaluate renal perfusion in critical illness. Indeed, it can be performed at the bedside, is minimally invasive and safe. Contrast-enhanced ultrasound provides information on the microcirculation and, potentially, could improve our understanding of flow alterations in critical illness associated AKI.

At present, imaging diagnostic tools are still in validation studies and offer only limited bedside support for the diagnosis of AKI.

5.5.**Biomarkers**. In the AKI biomarkers can be components of serum or urine. The term biomarker (acronym for biological marker) was first described in 1989, which means measurable indicator for a specific biologic condition and for specific disease process. In 2001, biomarker definition was standardized to be a characteristic that can be measured and evaluated as a normal biological process, pathological process, or pharmacological response to therapeutic intervention. Moreover, the Food Drug and Administration (FDA) uses the biomarker term to describe any diagnostic indicator that can be measured and used to assess any risk or disease. An ideal AKI biomarker should be accurate, reliable, easy to measure with a standard assay, non-invasive, reproducible and sensitive and specific with defined cutoff values. Urine represents an ideal body fluid for AKI biomarker assessment as it can be obtained noninvasively and repeatedly from a spontaneously voided sample or from an indwelling bladder catheter. The road to AKI biomarker validation spans discovery in pre-clinical studies from bodily fluids, assay development, retrospective study in completed trials and then prospective screening in ongoing trials. These phases must be completed before a biomarker can be used broadly in clinical practice. Conventional biochemical markers of AKI such as plasma creatinine accumulate in the blood as glomerular filtration rate (GFR) falls [Uchino 2010]. While creatinine changes remain the standard for diagnosis of AKI [3], plasma creatinine has many limitations [4]. Serum creatinine (SCr) is a degradation product of muscle cells and represents a surrogate for the efficiency of glomerular filtration. It has poor predictive accuracy for renal injury, particularly, in the early stages of AKI [Waikar et al., 2009]. In the case of critical illness, SCr concentrations are subject to large fluctuations due to a patient's induced dilutional volume status, the catabolic effects of critical illness, the

12

likelihood of concentration decreases in septic conditions and the increased tubular excretion with diminishing renal function. Furthermore, after an injurious event, the rise in SCr is slow. Therefore, detection of the earliest evidence of AKI necessitates the use of other plasma or urinary biomarkers.

5.5.1.**Plasma/serum cystatin C** (CyC). Cystatin C (CyC) is a 13-kDa non-glycosylated cysteine protease inhibitor produced by all nucleated cells at a constant rate. In healthy subjects, plasma CyC (pCyC) is excreted through glomerular filtration and metabolized completely by the proximal tubules. CyC can be measured in a random sample of serum. All measures are based on liquid agglutination of latex particles coated with polyclonal antibodies against CyC. which is coated on latex particles, and causes agglutination. The degree of the turbidity caused by agglutination can be measured optically and is proportional to the amount of CyC in the sample. There are two methods, depending on the nature of the signal measurement. Particle-enhanced turbidimetry immunoassay (PETIA) measures the transmitted light and Particle-enhanced nephelometric immunoassay (PENIA) measures the diffused light. Reference values may differ inmany populations, with sex and age. Across different studies, the mean reference interval (as defined by the 5th and 95th percentiles) was between 0,52 and 0,98 mg/L [Croda-Todd et al., 2007]. For women, the average reference interval is 0,52 to 0,90 mg/L with a mean of 0,71 mg/L. For men, the average reference interval is 0,56 to 0,98 mg/L with a mean of 0,77 mg/L. The normal values decrease until the first year of life, remaining relatively stable before they increase again, especially beyond age 50, Because of its constant rate of production, pCyC concentration is determined by glomerular filtration. pCyC is not diagnostically specific for AKI because it is an early marker of glomerular dysfunction rather than of tubular. Cystatin C in the sample binds to anti-cystatin C antibody, Furthermore, there is no evident tubular secretion. Several studies claim the superiority of pCyC against SCr to detect minor reductions in glomerular filtration rate [Dharnidharka et al., 2002]. However, the interpretation of pCyC levels is biased by older age, gender, weight, height, cigarette smoking and high levels of C-reactive protein [Okura et al., 2010]. In addition, CyC levels are supposedly influenced by abnormal thyroid function [Manelli et al., 2005], the use of immunosuppressive therapy and malignancies [Keller et al., 2007]. In 318 patients included at ICU admission, pCyC predicted developing sustained AKI (n=19) very modestly (area under the curve [AUC]=0,65 [95% confidence interval (CI) 0,58–0,71] in univariate analysis [Nejat et al., 2010]. Herget-Rosenthal et al. [2004] described a cohort in whom sCyC was measured at admission in 85 patients with normal GFR. The reported AUC was 0,82 (CI 0,71–0,92) for acute renal failure 2 days prior to the event. A recent multicenter study in 151 subjects in a comparative setting found a poorer performance (AUC=0,72 no CI provided) [Royakkers et al., 2004]. Metzger et al., [2010] compared the classification performance of a set of urinary proteome analyses with sCyC in 20 general ICU patients, retrospectively, and found low classification accuracy (AUC=0,67 CI. In cardio pulmonary bypass (CPB) cohorts, several studies explored the use of CyC for AKI prediction. Haase-Fielitz et al., [2009] described 100 cardiac surgical patients among whom 23 subjects were classified as patients without preoperative renal impairment. Their samples were measured at ICU arrival, and the reported AUC=0,78 (CI 0,58–0,99) did not improve after 24 h. Koyner et al., (2008) reported on 72 patients who were admitted following CPB with 34 subjects developing AKI, which was defined as a 25% increase in sCr or the need for RRT (n=7) within 3 days after surgery. SCyC measured at the time of ICU arrival was not a useful early predictor for the composite outcome AUC=0,62 (0,49–0,75) [Koyner et al., 2008]. A likely explanation is the applied unusual definition of AKI, which indicates less severe grades of AKI among the event group. Serum cystatin C levels increased with 82% sensitivity and 95% specificity 1,5 days earlier than serum creatinine in 44 patients who developed AKI. Using the outcomes of death or the need for renal replacement therapy, biomarkers have been tested for predictive efficacy. Serum cystatin C levels were 76% sensitive and 93% specific for renal replacement therapy (RRT) need 24 hours prior to initiation based on creatinine levels [Harget-Rosenthal et al., 2004]. In a number of baseline pediatric studies, serum cystatin C levels were diagnostically superior to serum creatinine and were independent of gender, body composition, or muscle mass [Zaffanello et al., 2007]

5.5.2.**Urine cystatin C**. The urinary excretion of CyC (uCyC) specifically reflects tubular damage because systemically produced cystatin C is normally not found in urine [Herget-Rosenthal et al., 2004]. However, recent insights show that urinary CyC excretion is augmented by albuminuria [Nejat et al., 2011]. In patients without AKI on ICU entry, uCyC was not predictive of AKI occurring within 48 h with AUC=0,54 (CI 0,46–0,62) [Nejat et al., 2010, Liangos et al., 2009] used uCyC for this prediction, which resulted in very moderate performances 2-h post-CPB surgery with ROC AUC=0,50 (CI 0,27–0,72) in a cohort of 103 patients with 13 events of AKI. In a study in patients undergoing CPB, Koyner et al. [2008] demonstrated that uCyC measured at ICU admission reached a maximum performance with an AUC of 0,693 (CI 0,567–0,818) [21,

14

48]. Among general adult ICU patients, 82 subjects developed AKI within 48 h of admission and the predictive performance for urine CyC corrected for urinary creatinine concentration yielded AUC=0,55 (CI 0,48–0,63). For the prediction of AKIN Stage 3 versus the rest of the cohort, the predictive performance increased to AUC=0,84 (CI 0,68–0,99) [Koyner et al., 2010]. Royakkers et al., [2011] regarded uCyC as a predictor for AKI 2 days prior to the first day of AKI and found no diagnostic value (AUC $\geq$ 0,49 no CI provided).

5.5.3.**Neutrophil gelatinase-associated lipocalin**. Neutrophil gelatinase-associated lipocalin (NGAL) is a small protein linked to neutrophil gelatinase in specific leukocyte granules [Borregaard et al., 1995]. It is also expressed in a variety of epithelial tissues associated with anti-microbial defence [Goetz et al., 2002]. In the normal kidney, only the distal tubules and collecting ducts stain for NGAL expression. NGAL's composite molecule binds ferric siderophores, and furthermore, it is a potent epithelial growth inducer, has protective effects in ischaemia [Mishra et al., 2004] and is up-regulated by systemic bacterial infections [Shapiro et al., 2009]. In the case of AKI, proximal tubule cells also stain for NGAL proteins, which is explained by megalin– cubilin-mediated re-uptake of NGAL present in the glomerular filtrate [Mori et al., 2005]. Urinary NGAL originates from local production in the distal tubules and collectiing ducts. However, uNGAL excretion is proportional to albumin excretion in mouse models of diabetic nephropathy and is thus augmented when the proximal transport maximum is exceeded. Siew et al., [2009] enrolled their patients within 24 h after admission and reported a receiver operating characteristic curve (ROC) AUC=0,77 (CI 0,64–0,90) for developing AKI in a subgroup of patients with estimated glomerular filtration rate (eGFR) at admission $\geq$75 mL/min/1,73 m^2 for urine NGAL (n=18, patients having AKI versus 257 patients without AKI). Cruz et al., [2010] reported on the development of AKI within 48 h after first sampling an AUC=0,78 (CI 0,65–0,90). However, the reported positive predictive value was low (24%), and within 5 days, the AUC was reduced to 0,67 (CI 0,55– 0,79) [Cruz et al., 2010]. The first sampling was performed within 24 h after ICU admission. De Geus et al., [2011] came to roughly similar reports with samples at ICU admission in patients with eGFR >60 mL/min/1,73 m^2 for both plasma and uNGAL AUC=0,75 ±[standard error (SE)] 0,103 AUC NGAL=0,79 ±(SE) 0,085. It is debatable whether the exclusion of patients with eGFR's <75 or 60 mL/min/1,73 m^2 applied by Siew and de Geus et al., is useful in clinical practice because a biomarker should also be effective in patients with CKD. In patients with sepsis, the predictive performance for

AKI seemed not to be affected, as reported by Martensson for both plasma and urine NGAL [respectively, AUCs=0,85 (CI 0,67–1,0) and 0,86 (CI 0,68–1,0)]; [Martensson et al., 2010]. Several studies report results in CPB cohorts: Koyner et al., [2010] measured both pNGAL AUC=0,526 (0,388–0,664) and uNGAL AUC=0,705 (CI 0,581–0,829) at ICU admission. An additional analysis by the same authors stratified their patients according to attained RIFLE stage and reported increased performances when using the harder end point of failure AUC=0,69 (0,57–0,80) and AKIN Stage 3 AUC=0,79 (0,65–0,94) [Koyner et al., 2010]. A large study (n=426) in CPB patients demonstrated test performance association with the pre-surgery baseline eGFR. Interestingly, only in patients with an eGFR above 60mL/min was NGAL predictive: AUC=0,68 (CI 0,54–0,81) [McIlroy et al., 2010]. A much smaller study (n=9 events) reported values for both pNGAL and uNGAL, corrected for urinary creatinine: AUC=0,85 (CI 0,73–0,97) and AUC=0,96 (CI 0,90–1,0), respectively [Tuladhar et al., 2009]. Haase-Fielitz [2009] compared the performance of conventional and novel markers for pNGAL in adult CPB patients, excluding patients with preoperative renal impairment NGAL: the results yielded AUC=0,80 (CI 0,58–0,99). Wagener et al., [2008] performed a study in adult CPB patients: for urine NGAL, the predictive performance was AUC=0,573 (CI 0,506–0,640) directly after the operation and the performance increased until 18 h after ICU admission to a maximum of 0,611. These results were similar also in 103 CPB patients 2 h after surgery: AUC=0,50 (CI 0,33–0,68) [Liangos et al., 2009]. Among general adult ICU patients, 82 subjects developed AKI within 48 h of admission, and the predictive performance for NGAL corrected for urinary creatinine concentration yielded AUC=0,55 (CI 0,48–0,63) (Endre et al., 2011) [Endre et al., 2011]. Metzger et al., (2010) compared the classification performance of urinary proteome analysis with classical markers. For urine NGAL, the ROC analysis revealed low classification accuracy: AUC=0,54 CI (not provided) [Metzger et al., 2010]. The only meta-analysis published to date assessed pNGAL's ability to predict across different settings; when weighted for study sample size, this value yielded an overall AUC of 0,782 (CI 0,689–0,872) [Haase et al., 2009]. In pediatrics, uNGAL levels demonstrated sharp increases to >5000 ng/mg within 2-4 hours in patients who would eventually require RRT [Bennett et al., 2008]. Urinary NGAL (uNGAL) levels of ≥ 50 µg/L were 100% sensitive and 98% predictive in the 20/71 children post CPB who developed AKI [Mishra et al., 2005]. In a prospective cohort study, mean and peak uNGAL concentrations rose at least six-fold higher in children with AKI than control patients admitted to the PICU (26). Serum NGAL levels within 2 hours

16

of PB of ≥ 150 mg/L were 84% sensitive and 94% predictive in children who developed AKI within 3 days [Dent et al., 2007]. Additionally, the uNGAL area under the receiver operating curve for predicting worsening of AKI was 0,61. Recently, a number of early markers of AKI have been identified from proteomic analysis of plasma and urine from patients who go on to develop AKI [Ichimura et al., 1998]. By identifying substances that change in concentration early in the time course of AKI, diagnosis may be accelerated and additional insights into the pathogenesis of kidney injury obtained.

5.5.4.**Interleukin-18 (IL-18).** Interleukin-18 is a proinflammatory cytokine of the IL-1 superfamily. It is synthesized in an inactive form by several tissues including monocytes, macrophages, and proximal tubular epithelial cells. In animal models the role of IL-18 was demonstrated in postischemic AKI. Studies of isolated mouse proximal tubules demonstrated elevation of IL-18 following hypoxia, and mice with ischemic AKI had increased urinary levels of IL-18 [Edelstein et al., 2007]. The ability of IL-18 to mediate ischemic proximal tubular injury in mice has led to the assumption that it can be used as an early biomarker of AKI in humans. IL-18 is measured through ELISA or a specific assay for their detection. In animal models, IL-18 has proven to be an important mediator in the process of AKI. Therefore, its urinary release has been anticipated as a possible early marker: several studies have explored the clinical application of this hypothesis. Among general adult ICU patients, 82 subjects developed AKI within 48 h of admission, and the predictive performance for IL-18 corrected for urinary creatinine concentration was AUC=0,55 (CI 0,47–0,62) [Edre et al., 2011]. Metzger et al., [2010] compared the classification performance of urinary proteome analysis with classical markers. For urine IL-18, the ROC analysis revealed low classification accuracy (AUC=0,57). Nevertheless, in a large cohort of mixed patients (n=451), Siew et al., [2010] enrolled patients within 24 h after ICU admission: 86 developed AKI. The overall predictive performance reported was AUC=0,62 (CI 0,54–0,69); this value increased slightly in patients with an eGFR above 75 mL/min/1,73 m^2 [AUC=0,67 (CI 0,53–0,81)]. There seemed to be a strong association with sepsis. In patients with acute lung injury, uIL-18 predicted progression to AKI within 24 h with an accuracy of AUC=0,731 (CI not provided) with substantial overlap between cases and controls in urine concentrations [Parikh et al., 2005]. In CPB patients, 2 hr after CPB time, the optimal performance was reported to yield an AUC=0,66 (CI 0,49–0,83).

5.5.5.**Liver fatty acid binding protein.** (L-FABP) Fatty acid binding proteins are small (15 kDa) cytoplasmatic proteins abundantly expressed in tissues with active fatty acid metabolism. Their primary function is the facilitation of long-chain fatty acid transport, the regulation of gene expression and the reduction of oxidative stress. Urinary liver fatty acid binding protein (L-FABP) is undetectable in healthy control urine, which is explained by efficient proximal tubular internalization via megalin-mediated endocytosis [Oyama et al., 2005]. Under ischaemic conditions, tubular L-FABP gene expression is induced; in renal disease, the proximal tubular re-absorption of L-FABP is reduced [Yamamoto et al., 2007]. Urinary L-FABP is measured by enzyme-linked immunosorbent assay (ELISA). To date, there is one small study reporting on the early diagnostic performance of L-FABP in adult ICU patients. The reported ROC AUC value was 0,95, no CI provided. However, several uncertainties remain after disclosure of the study's methodology. Firstly, patient selection (n=25 with 14 AKI and 11 non-AKI) seems to have been a result of convenient sampling. Secondly, the "true early diagnosis" remains very doubtful as peak SCr and L-FABP values are reported as having the same median value; no further clear information concerning timing is provided [Matsui et al., 2011]. In the in the case control study of 27 post-CPB surgery pediatric patients [Ivanišević et al., 2013] find significant differences between patients with and without AKI in L-FABP levels at 2, 6, and 48 h after surgery, length of hospital stay, and CPB time; L-FABP was normalized to urinary creatinine concentration at all time points, with area under the receiver operator curve (AUC ROC) 0,867 at 2 and 6 h postoperatively. Correlation coefficient between L-FABP and length of hospital stay after surgery was statistically significant (r = 0,722, p value = 0,000).

5.5.6.**Kidney injury molecule-1**. Kidney injury molecule-1 (KIM-1) is a Type I transmembrane glycoprotein with a cleavable ectodomain (90 kDa) which is localized in the apical membrane of dilated tubules in acute and chronic injury [Baily et al., 2002]. KIM-1 is believed to play a role in regeneration processes after epithelial injury and in the removal of dead cells in the tubular lumen through phagocytosis [Bonventre, 2009]. A reduction in proteinuria with renine angiotensin aldosteron blockade is accompanied by a reduction in urinary KIM-1 excretion [Waanders et al., 2010]. Among general adult ICU patients, 82 subjects developed AKI within 48 h of admission, and the predictive performance for KIM-1 corrected for urinary creatinine concentration yielded AUC=0,55 (CI 0,47–0,62) in the study of Endre et al., [2011]. Metzger et al., [2010] compared the classification performance of urinary proteome analysis with classical markers. For urine KIM-1, the ROC analysis revealed low classification accuracy (AUC=0,71 CI, not provided) [Mezger et al., 2010]. Several studies report its diagnostic properties in adult

CPB patients. Liang et al., [2010] reported an AUC for progressive AKI of 0,69 (CI 0,61–0,78) after 6 h of inclusion. Notably, adding KIM-1 to interleukin (IL)-18 [AUC for IL-18 for progressive AKI 6 h after inclusion was 0,87 (CI 0,80–0,93)] in a predictive model improved the model's accuracy only minimally [AUC 0,88 (CI 0,82–0,93)]. Liangos et al., [2009] reported an AUC 2-h post- CPB surgery of 0,78 (CI 0,64–0,91): however, in multivariate regression analysis, the association of KIM-1 was attenuated after adjustment. Koyner et al., [2010] found an AUC 0,56 (CI 0,45–0,67) as admission value for the entire cohort with an improvement when predicting AKIN Stage 3 only [AUC ≥0,69 (CI 0,44–0,93)]. Parikh et al., in the multicenter cohort study involving 1219 adults and 311 children shows that KIM-1 levels peaked 2 days after surgery in adults and 1 day after surgery in children. KIM-1 levels remained significantly elevated compared with the non-AKI group until day 5 in the adult AKI group and day 4 in the pediatric AKI group. After multivariable adjustment, higher KIM-1 and L-FABP were associated with a longer length of stay in the ICU and in the hospital for both adults and children (adjusted P for trend <0,001 in adults and adjusted P for trend <0,001 in children [Parikh et al., 2005].

5.5.7.**Urinary hepcidin**. Recently, urinary hepcidin has been suggested as a candidate biomarker of AKI [Ho et al., 2009]. In particular, the active form of hepcidin (hepcidin-25) may increase in the urine on the day after surgery in patients not developing AKI after cardiac surgery [9]. This inverse association between urinary hepcidin and post CPB AKI may be a unique feature of hepcidin as a biomarker [Prowle et al., 2010] in comparison with more established biomarkers of AKI, such as neutrophil gelatinase-associated lipocalin (NGAL) that are positively correlated with AKI [8]. No quantitative information, however, exists on the relationship between urinary hepcidin, the urinary hepcidin:creatinine ratio and the fractional excretion (FE) of hepcidin after CPB and subsequent AKI. Authors find that urinary hepcidin and hepcidin: creatinine ratio may be an early post-operative biomarker of AKI after CPB with an inverse association between postopertive urinary hepcidin concentrations and risk and severity of subsequent AKI. Our results indicate that elevated urinary hepcidin concentration and urinary hepcidin: creatinine ratios at 24 h post-CPB surgery are informative biomarkers of healthy renal function in patients who will not develop AKI.

5.5.8.**Biomarkers summary**. Acute kidney injury is a clinical situation with increased morbidity and mortality, especially among the ICU patients. Detection of AKI with current RIFLE and AKIN criteria is based on the increase in serum creatinine or decrease in urine output. Serum creatinine is unreliable and delayed marker of kidney damage.

Serum creatinine becomes abnormal when more than 50% of GFR is lost, and it takes up to 24 hours before increases in blood concentration are detectable. New biomarkers, such as neutrophil gelatinase associated lipocalin (NGAL), cystatin C (CyC), kidney injury molecule-1 (KIM-1), interleukin-18 (IL-18) and liver type fatty acid binding protein (L-FABP), seem to be more efficient in detecting AKI before the rise in serum creatinine. However various clinical studies of novel biomarkers have demonstrated moderate diagnostic accuracy. The majority of the studies reported were from single centers that enrolled small numbers of subjects and until now there are no determinant cutoff values for either of the new biomarkers. Clinical applications of various biomarkers are summarized in the Table 5.

Table 5.   **Application of various biomarkers for diagnosis of AKI**

Neutrophil gelatinase-associated lipocalin (NGAL)	Prediction of AKI: •Post-cardiopulmonary bypass surgery •After contrast exposure •In sepsis •In trauma patients •In critically ill adult patients •In delayed graft function after renal transplantation Prediction of: •Progression of AKI •Duration and severity of AKI and length of stay in ICU •Adverse outcomes in patients with AKI •Need for RRT •Mortality in patients on RRT •Need for RRT or death after cardiac surgery •Severity of AKI and need for RRT in patients in the emergency department •Recovery of AKI after pneumonia •GFR in patients with chronic kidney disease Differentiation between transient and sustained AKI in adults on admission to ICU, and between 'pre-renal' and intrinsic AKI

Cystatin C	Prediction of AKI: •In critically ill adults •Post-cardiac surgery •In liver transplant recipients •Post-coronary angiography •In critically ill patients with baseline estimated GFR <60 ml/minute Prediction of: Severity and duration of AKI and length of ICU stay post-cardiac surgery •RRT in critically ill patients, post-cardiac surgery and in patients with AKI seen by nephrology consult service Correlation with AKI post-cardiac surgery No improved prediction of AKI in adult renal transplant recipients or ICU patients
IL-18	Prediction of AKI: •After renal transplantation •Post-cardiac surgery •In patients with acute lung injury •In critically ill patients Prediction of: •14-day mortality in critically ill patients Progression of AKI •Need for RRT or death after cardiac surgery •Mortality in patients with acute lung injury
Kidney injury molecule-1 (KIM-1)	Prediction of AKI: •Post-cardiac surgery •In critically ill patients •In patients with AKI seen by nephrology consult service •In critically ill patients with baseline estimated GFR <60 ml/minute Prediction of adverse outcome in hospitalized patients with AKI

Liver-type fatty acid binding protein (L-FABP)	Prediction of: •AKI in critically ill patients •Poor outcome in patients with AKI •AKI post coronary angiography
Hepcidin	Correlation between lower urinary hepcidin levels and AKI post-cardiac surgery

6.Management of AKI.

Development of management parameters in AKI is limited by the multifactorial etiology of the disease process and by the paucity of prospectively validated data.

6.1.Fluid replacement strategies.

Fluid resuscitation is a common practice in critically ill patients. In AKI patients, it is difficult to assess fluid requirements due to the multifactorial nature of AKI, the limited accuracy of current diagnostic techniques to determine volume status [Antonelli et al., 2006] and the absence of practical tests to quantify renal blood flow. However, overly aggressive fluid replacement is often deleterious and associated with an increased risk of mortality, as demonstrated in two studies published in 2011 [Myburg et al., 2011; Arikan et al., 2011]. Maitland et al. performed a randomized trial with children in subsaharian Africa who suffered from shock and life-threatening infections [Matland et al. 2011]. The trial was stopped early because fluid resuscitation with albumin or saline was associated with increased 48- hour mortality in children with impaired perfusion. Boyd et al. investigated the effects of a positive fluid balance in adult patients with septic shock both early in resuscitation and after 4 days [Boyd et al. 2011]. Authors found that a strongly positive fluid balance is associated with increased risk of mortality. However, best survival in these patients was seen with a moderately positive fluid balance of approximately 3 liters at 12 hours., these analyses suggest that positive fluid balance may be deleterious in sepsis as well as in AKI and should be dealt with promptly. Although volume resuscitation might be required to maintain cardiac output, the resultant fluid accumulation can considerably contribute to organ dysfunction, particularly in patients with AKI. A novel conceptual framework for fluid management in critical illness introduces the idea of interrelated phases of fluid management differentiated according to the clinical status of the patient with evolving goals for fluid need [Arikan et al. 2012]. The model proposed for the epidemiology of fluid balance in AKI may be extended across the spectrum of critical illness with caveats: (A) In the initial phase of acute resuscitation- the objective is restoration of effective circulating blood volume, organ perfusion and tissue oxygenation. Fluid accumulation and a positive fluid balance may be expected; (B) In the second phase of resuscitation-the goal is maintenance of intravascular volume homeostasis. The objective during this phase is to prevent excessive fluid accumulation and avoid unnecessary fluid loading; and (C) In the final stage, the objective centers around fluid removal and the concept of active "de-resuscitation" coresponding to a state of physiologic stabilization, organ injury recovery and convalescence. During this phase, unnecessary fluid accumulation may contribute to secondary organ injury and adverse events. Numerous studies in perioperative and critical care settings support this concept of "ebb and flow" in fluid loading, fluid accumulation and removal. Indeed, these phases of resuscitation likely exist on a continuum and the observed variability in fluid balance is understood to be a dynamic process, does not necessarily follow a fixed temporal pattern or time scale and is likely highly individualized. For example, in septic patients with acute lung injury, the balance between early goal-directed therapy aimed at adequate initial fluid resuscitation coupled with downstream diuretic use and "de-resuscitation" (*i.e.*, conservative late fluid management) can improve outcomes [Myburg et al. 2007]. Similarly in pediatric septic shock, outcome improved with early appropriate fluid therapy [Gattas et al. 2013]. Such phasic need for fluid and then need for active fluid removal has also been demonstrated in perioperative settings [Hercog et al., 2012]. Inappropriate fluid therapy, regardless of fluid type, may disrupt compensatory mechanisms and worsen outcome. In patients with sepsis-associated AKI, continued fluid loading in the setting of apparent optimal systemic hemodynamics was shown not to improve kidney function, but worsen lung function and oxygenation [Arikan et al. 2012].

6.2. Crystalloids or colloids?

In the adult population, studies have compared Albumin to saline (SAFE study) and hydroxyethylstarches to saline (SOAP study) [Finfer et al., 2004] for resuscitation. Neither demonstrated clear benefit in colloid over crystalloid infusions. There was no survival difference in >7,000 patients between recipients of albumin or saline (SAFE study). They has found fluid accumulation to be a predictor of 60-day mortality (HR = 1,21/L per 24 h, 95%CI: 1,13-1,28; $P < 0.001$) [Finfer et al. 2004]. However, in three randomized studies of children with severe malaria, albumin conferred a survival advantage when compared with both normal saline and gelatin [Akech et al., 2006, 2010; Maitland et al., 2005].

6.3. Role of fluid balance.

No consensus exists regarding the appropriate balance of fluids, diuresis, and RRT to use in AKI. In response to hypoperfusion, many patients may receive total fluid doses to reach central venous pressure and mean arterial pressure targets that result in total body water overload. Pediatric studies have pioneered the concept now well established in all ages that fluid overload is an independent risk factor for mortality in AKI. The Prospective Pediatric Continuous Renal Replacement Therapy Registry Group

24

(Prospective Pediatric CRRT), studying a sample of 116 children, retrospectively found increased fluid administration to be independently associated with mortality in children started on CRRT [Goldstein et al., 2005]. When Goldstein et al. [Goldstein et al., 2001] first published on the potential detrimental effects of cumulative fluid overload, there was a lot of resistance from the critical care community about their conclusions as there was new data on the importance of aggressive goal-directed use of fluids in the early course of sepsis [de Oliveira et al., 2008].

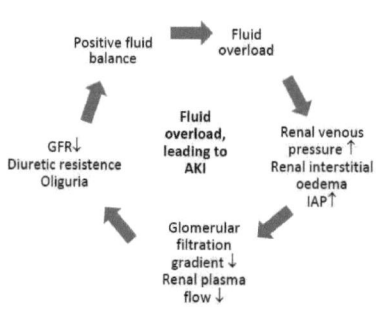

Fig. 1.   Vitious circle of fluid overload

In pediatrics, the percent fluid overload has been used as an initiating trigger and is calculated as follows: fluid overload=[(Fluids IN +fluids OUT) /admission weight] ×100. In a study of 113 children with multiple organ dysfunction syndrome started on CRRT, median percent fluid overload was significantly lower in survivors compared to nonsurvivors (7,8% vs. 15,1%), independent of severity of illness [Foland et al., 2004]. A recent analysis of 340 children [Sutherland et al., 2010] used a tripartite classification for percent fluid overload at initiation of renal replacement therapy: < 10%, 10–20%, and ≥20% fluid overload. Those with ≥20% fluid overload had a 66% mortality rate, whereas those with 10–20% fluid overload displayed a lower mortality rate of 43%, and those with <10% fluid overload had the lowest mortality rate of 29%. The association between degree of fluid overload and mortality remained after adjusting for intergroup differences and severity of illness [Sutherland et al., 2010]. Patients with ≥20% fluid overload had an 8.5-fold greater adjusted odds ratio of death than those with <20% fluid overload.

6.4.**Intraabdominal hypertension.**

A mechanism by which fluid overload may contribute directly to renal dysfunction is by leading to intra-abdominal hypertension (IAH) and the abdominal compartment syndrome (ACS), both of which are associated with significant morbidity and mortality in critically ill patients. The kidneys are vulnerable to even small increases in IAP, and oliguria is one of the first visible signs of IAH. Inadequate renal perfusion pressure and renal filtration gradient (FG) have been proposed as key factors in the development of IAP-induced renal failure [De laet et al., 2007]. The FG is the mechanical force across the glomerulus and equals the difference between the glomerular filtration pressure

25

(GFP) and the proximal tubular pressure (PTP). In the presence of IAH, GFP may be approximated as MAP minus IAP (or APP) while PTP may be assumed to equal IAP. The FG is thus defined as MAP minus two times the IAP, illustrating that changes in IAP have a greater impact upon renal function and urine production than do changes in MAP. Elevated IAP leads to compression of intra-abdominal vessels, compromised microvascular blood flow, and increased renal venous pressure, which in turn results in impaired renal plasma flow, decreased glomerular filtration rate, and oliguria (Fig. 1). Preventing fluid overload and rapid correction of fluid overload with early initiation of renal replacement therapy may represent "low-hanging" fruits in pediatric AKI therapeutics that deserve investigation. Prompt recognition, often guided by urinary bladder pressure measurement, and surgical treatment offer the best potential for recovery.

6.5.Maintaining Renal Perfusion.

In the acute setting, the two most significant threats to renal perfusion pressure are systemic arterial hypotension and increased intra-abdominal pressure (including so-called abdominal compartment syndrome). Specific recommendations to maintain renal perfusion are difficult to make. First, vasopressor medications (e.g. norepinephrine) should be used only to treat arterial hypotension once intravascular volume has been restored. In practice, vasopressors are often started as volume loading is underway and discontinued if no longer required, once hypovolaemia has been reversed [Kellum, Pinsky, 2002]. Conventionally, a reduction in RBF and renal ischaemia have been regarded central to the pathogenesis of AKI in critical illness [Schrier, Wang, 2004]; however, the situation is likely to be more complex. In animal models, AKI has been reported when cardiac output was preserved or elevated [Langenberg et al. 2005], and subtotal (90%) occlusion of the renal arteries did not lead to prolonged AKI [Saotome et al., 2010]. Furthermore, cardiac arrest and warm renal ischaemia in humans only lead to significant AKI in the presence of severe post-resuscitation disease and cardiogenic shock [Chua et al., 2012]. These observations infer that local and systemic inflammatory responses, changes in intra-RBF distribution, microcirculatory dysfunction and glomerular haemodynamics may all account for loss of kidney function, even in the presence of maintained or increased RBF. Fluid administration has been shown to augment both cardiac output and RBF without an overall increase in renal oxygen delivery [Wan et al., 2007], while fluid resuscitation in an experimental model of haemorrhagic shock can restore blood pressure and cardiac output without recovery of

26

renal tissue oxygen tension [Legrand et al., 2010]. Finally, even when renal oxygen delivery is reduced, increased oxygen extraction may maintain renal oxygen consumption [Dyson et al., 2011] – suggesting that increasing renal oxygen delivery by increasing cardiac output may not avert AKI. To limit ischemic injury, attempts are made to modulate renal perfusion pressure and to optimize renal preload.

6.5.1.**Renal vasodilators**.The use of renal vasodilators to increase renal perfusion has not demonstrated improved outcomes. Adult studies of low-dose, or "renal-dose," dopamine have failed to show benefit and actually may even be harmful [Bellomo et al., 2000, Venkataraman et al. 2007]. Low-dose dopamine in children has not been effective at improving outcomes either [Andreoli, 2009]. A metaanalysis of dopamine use in adults showed that in 24 studies, dopamine did not prevent mortality (relative risk, 0,9 [0,44-1,83]), the onset of acute kidney failure (relative risk, 0,81 [0,55-1,19]), or the need for dialysis (relative risk, 0,83 [0,55-1,24]) [Kellum, 2001]. In another metaanalysis of 61 trials, low dose dopamine increased urine output by 24% but resulted in no significant improvement in serum creatinine levels [Friedrich et al., 2005]. Low dose dopamine in children has not been effective at improving outcomes either [Filler, 2001]. Further, low dose dopamine may increase the risk of tachyarrhythmias and ischemic injury to the myocardium by increasing myocardial oxygen consumption. Additionally, its natriuretic effects may worsen the effective hypovolemia seen in AKI. Fenoldopam, a selective dopamine agonist, increases renal blood flow and may reduce mortality and the need for RRT in adults but has not significantly improved AKI outcomes in children [Ricci et al., 2008]. Compared to low dose dopamine, fenoldopam dosed from 0,05 to 0,1 µg/kg/min was shown to improve serum creatinine values in 100 adults matched for severity of illness [Brienza et al., 2006], but showed no difference in 80 patients undergoing cardiac surgery [Bove et al., 2005]. Fenoldopam of $0,07 \leq 0,08$ mg/kg/min increased urine output in critically ill children with progressive oliguria [Moffet et al., 2008], but did not affect overall outcome. Neither low-dose dopamine nor fenoldopam have been tested in a large prospective cohort pediatric study and cannot be recommended for prevention or management of AKI outside of the context of a clinical trial. Kidney is a highly adaptive organ designed to maintain renal perfusion and GFR over a wide range of blood pressures.

6.5.2.**Optimization of systemic blood pressure**. Autoregulatory mechanisms are first line of defense, however, maybe significantly impaired: a) as a consequence of: underlying kidney disease and b) as a consequence of AKI secondary to drug therapy.

Maintaining an adequate filtration pressure gradient is key to maintaining GFR. Many clinicians and clinical protocols target a mean arterial pressure of 60–65 mmHg. However, patients with long-standing hypertension and/or renal vascular disease may require substantially higher pressures to maintain renal perfusion. Restoration of MAP from 60 to 75 mmHg improves renal oxygen delivery, GFR and the renal oxygen supply/demand relationship in post-cardiac surgery patients with vasodilatory shock and AKI. This pressure-dependent renal perfusion, filtration and oxygenation at levels of MAP below 75 mmHg reflect a more or less exhausted renal autoregulatory reserve [Redfors et al., 2011]. In critically ill patients, one study in 217 patients found a MAP of up to 82 mmHg may be required to prevent AKI [Badin et al. 2011]. Similarly, a study in 31 critically ill patients demonstrated periods with a systolic blood pressure less than 90 mmHg for at least 30 min were associated with higher levels of cardiac enzymes. One study performed in patients undergoing noncardiac surgery found that in those who were at high risk for AKI, periods of a MAP less than 60 mmHg were more common in those who developed AKI than those who did not [Kheterpal et al., 2009]. Furthermore, using classification and regression tree analysis, Bijker et al.[2009] found a MAP less than 50 mmHg had the largest independent association with death in their study in 1705 patients undergoing noncardiac surgery. In human septic shock, two interventional prospective studies of limited size [LeDoux et.al., 2000; Bourgoin et al., 2005] have shown that increasing MAP from 65 to 75 or 85 mmHg with norepinephrine did not result in urinary output nor serum creatinine significant improvement. There is no evidence from clinical studies or appropriately designed animal experiments [Langenberg et al., 2005] that norepinephrine is associated with increased risk of AKI when used to treat arterial hypotension. Indeed, a large observational study [Sakr et al., 2006], suggest that other vasopressors, dopamine, may be less efficacious and possibly associated with lower survival. Conversely, in another recent study [Deruddre et al. 2007], increasing MAP from 65 to 75 mmHg resulted in an increase in urinary output in 11 septic shock patients. Further, a recent retrospective cohort study suggested that levels of MAP higher than 75 mmHg could be necessary to insure renal protection during sepsis and septic shock [Dunser et al., 2009]. Current recommendations for the prevention of AKI in the ICU [Joanidis et al., 2010] propose to achieve a MAP above 60 to 65 mmHg but indicate that this target pressure should be individualized when possible, especially if knowledge of the premorbid blood pressure is available. In case of chronic hypertension, the autoregulation MAP thresholds are known to be higher than in normotensive patients, and

28

this could suggest that higher levels of blood pressure are necessary in hypertensive patients to maintain RBF [Abuelo, 2007]. Aronson et al. [2008] reported that the magnitude and duration of systolic blood pressure excursions outside of predefined limits (65 to 135 mmHg intraoperatively, 75 to 145 mmHg pre- and postoperatively) predicted cardiac surgery-associated AKI. A difference in preoperative and average MAP during CPB >26 mmHg was further found to be independently associated with cardiac surgery-associated AKI [Hogue et al., 2006]. These results indicate that raising MAP targets during CPB might reduce the frequency of postoperative AKI. Preoperative pulse pressure has been identified previously as a risk factor for AKI after cardiac surgery with CPB [Borodka et al., 2011]. Kanji et al. [2010] found that pulse pressure > 60 mmHg was more common in those who developed AKI than in those who did not. Elevated pulse pressure indicates central vascular stiffness, which may lead to arteriolar narrowing that necessitates higher blood pressure for renal perfusion during surgery. These data are valid in adult patients, in children, according the PALS guidelines [Pediatric Advanced Life Support, 2000], *hypotension* is characterized by the following: For term neonates (0 to 28 days of age), SBP <60 mm Hg, for infants from 1 month to 12 months, SBP <70 mm Hg, for children >1 year to 10 years, SBP <70+(2×age in years), beyond 10 years, hypotension is defined as an SBP <90 mm Hg. Consensus among pediatric anesthetists regarding the definition of intraoperative hypotension is still lacking [Naftiu et al., 2007] and a specific arterial pressure targets for titration of therapy to avoid renal hypoperfusion are not known.

6.6.**Diuretics**.

The physiological rationale for using diuretics in AKI begins with maintaining urine flow. In theory, urine flow flushes out debris, including denuded epithelium, and avoids tubular obstruction and back leak of glomerular filtrate into the renal interstitium, which further perpetuates renal injury. Furthermore, given that some studies have shown that oliguric AKI carries a worse prognosis than nonoliguric AKI [Venkataraman, Kellum; 2005] many clinicians treat oliguria with diuretics. This line of reasoning has lead to the idea that maintaining an enhanced urinary flow in the setting of a renal insult is desirable. Loop diuretics also decrease the metabolic demand of the renal tubular cells and reduce their oxygen consumption. [Heyman et al., 1989]. Thus, these diuretic effects may theoretically protect the renal tubular cells from ischemia. Loop diuretics also reduce renal vascular resistance and may, therefore, increase renal blood flow (RBF), possibly by the inhibition of prostaglandin dehydrogenase [Ludens et al., 1968]. This inhibition leads to decreased degradation of PGE2, a potent renal vasodilator, which subsequently contributes to the increased RBF. All of the above theoretical advantages of loop diuretics, along with the prospect of easier management of fluid and electrolyte balance in patients with AKI, have lead to the widespread use of these drugs. Moreover, if AKI results in oliguria, diuretics are used to manage volume overload. Much of the controversy surrounding the use of diuretics in AKI stems from the conflict regarding the following two goals: prevention of renal injury and management of volume overload.

6.6.1.**Osmotic diuretics (mannitol)**. These agents are freely filtered at the glomerulus, undergo limited reabsorption by the renal tubule, and are relatively inert pharmacologically. They act primarily at the loop of Henle and also on the proximal tubule by extracting water from intracellular compartments. Osmotic diuretics expand the extracellular fluid volume, decrease blood viscosity, and inhibit renin release. These effects generally result in an increase in RBF and a reduction in medullary tonicity. The renal protection afforded by mannitol may be due to the removal of obstructing tubular casts, dilution of nephrotoxic substances in the tubular fluid, and/or reduction in the swelling of tubular elements *via* osmotic extraction of water. In addition, mannitol has also been shown to increase RBF and to act as a free-radical scavenger during reperfusion of the kidney. Although prophylactic mannitol is effective in animal models of ATN, the clinical efficacy of mannitol is less well established. Most published clinical studies have been underpowered and uncontrolled and shown conflicting results. Solomon et al., [1994] randomized 78 patients with mild to moderate renal insufficiency to receive either 0.45% saline alone, saline plus mannitol, In summary, despite the presence of animal and anecdotal human evidence for the beneficial effects of mannitol, there are no adequately powered, prospective, randomized clinical trials comparing these effects with those of saline hydration alone. Thus, mannitol cannot be scientifically justified in the prevention or management of AKI. The mannitol-induced increase in RVO$_2$ was, however, not matched by a proportional increase in RBF. Thus, a renal oxygen supply/demand mismatch was induced by mannitol in these postoperative patients. This was also reflected by the highly significant increase in renal oxygen extraction during mannitol infusion and the close relationship between FF and renal oxygen extraction. These findings are consistent with animal data which have shown that mannitol decreases outer medullary oxygen tension while cortical oxygen tension is unaffected Evans et al., 2000].

6.6.2. **Loop diuretics**. Loop diuretics (LD's) are frequently administered to critically ill children to manage the high fluid load that is prescribed daily and to control fluid balance. LD pharmacologic action is exerted at the thick ascending limb of Henle loop by reversibly blocking one of the chloride-binding sites of the $Na+/K+/2\ Cl-$ carrier. Consequently, reabsorption of filtered sodium is inhibited. Furosemide has also been shown to block the tubuloglomerular feedback response [Nishiyama et al., 2001]. There are three determinants of diuretic response to furosemide: the urinary concentrations of furosemide; the time of delivery of furosemide to the site of action; and the dynamics of the response at the site of action [Brater 1981].This intense natriuresis promotes an increased diuresis [Eades, Christensen ; 1998]. In Pediatric Intensive Care Units, LDs are routinely administered by either intermittent or continuous intravenous infusions [van der Vorst et al., 2001]. The vast majority of pediatric cardiac surgery patients receive LDs in the preoperative, intraoperative, and postoperative phases. LDs are the mainstay of therapy in children with congenital heart disease (CHD), particularly in the near-postoperative phase: they are essential for the management of fluid loading and the leak syndrome occurring after cardiopulmonary bypass (CPB) and of the high fluid administration needed for postoperative therapies and nutrition [Ricci et al., 2011]. Therefore, diuretics, are recommended for management of fluid overload in adults and children [Kellums et al., 2013]. Furthermore, in patients with cardiac dysfunction, LDs are needed both for left ventricular failure (to decrease hypervolemia, ventricular filling pressures, and pulmonary congestion) and right ventricular failure (to control fluid accumulation and systemic venous congestion, both of which are causes of renal and splanchnic organ dysfunction) [Felker et al., 2011]. The presence of well-known side effects, however, including metabolic alkalosis, the risk of neurohormonal activation, systemic vasoconstriction, electrolyte disturbances, impairment of renal function, and perhaps, worse clinical outcomes, may lead to arguments against an aggressive diuretic approach in these patients [Klinge, 2001]. It was previously shown that continuous infusion of furosemide causes a gradual increase in urine output (UO) that is significantly superior, in terms of total daily diuresis, to the unpredictable urine volume secondary to intermittent boluses [Luciani et al., 1997]. Current guidelines recommend using the minimum dose of LD required to keep the patient free of signs and symptoms of congestion [Jessup et al., 2009]. Although the once-daily use of furosemide might be convenient for some patients, it is not optimal from a pharmacodynamics perspective, since daily dosing results in a long period of sodium avidity by the kidney when therapeutic diuretic concentrations are not present. More frequent furosemide dosing serves to limit this "rebound" effect [Wittner et al., 1991]. Furosemide has been the most widely studied loop diuretic with regard to administration via continuous infusion in children [van der Vorst et al., 2006]. In a study by van der Vorst et al., [2], the authors suggested that continuous high-dose intravenous (IV) furosemide was well tolerated, safe, and effective in reducing volume overload in hemodynamically unstable infants after CPB surgery. The use of continuous infusion LD has attracted tremendous attention. This method has proven beneficial in patients with a diuretic resistance or tolerance to conventional intermittent therapy [Martin, Danzinger 1994]. Several potential advantages of continuous infusion LD have been identified, including decreased electrolyte loss secondary to a lower dosage of diuretic, production of a more reliable urine flow, and decreased alterations in fluid balance [Singh et al., 1992; Luciani et al., 1997] found that the administration of LD via continuous infusion produced a more controlled diuresis with less variation in hemodynamic parameters. Despite the wide use of furosemide and the fact that continuous infusion intuitively seems superior to bolus injections, evidence on this topic is still lacking. Meta-analysis showed that continuous infusion and bolus administration were associated with similar amounts of administered furosemide [Andoni et al., 2012]. Hager et al., compared low dose furosemide (1 mg/h) with placebo in 121 patients admitted to the ICU after major surgery. This work demonstrated that there was no difference in postoperative serum creatinine or creatinine clearance [Hager et al., 1996]. The most convincing study was performed in 126 cardiac surgery patients, randomized to receive either furosemide (0.5μg/kg/min), dopamine, or placebo, which were started at anesthesia induction. Compared with placebo, furosemide resulted not only in a significantly higher urine output but also in a more pronounced postoperative increase of serum creatinine [Lassingg, et al., 2000]. The authors concluded that furosemide was 'detrimental' and that its use was not superior to placebo (isotonic saline) for protection against renal dysfunction after cardiac surgery. However, despite this common use, there are no data to establish that loop diuretics have a beneficial effect on renal function. Radiocontrast administration is a leading cause of acute changes in renal function in hospitalized patients [Solomon et al., 1994]. Nevertheless, the pathogenesis of AKI in this setting is not completely understood. However, animal studies have suggested that loop diuretics could provide a benefit in this setting,6 and four prospective randomized clinical studies have evaluated the potential protective effects of loop diuretics in patients receiving radiocontrast [Dussol et al., 2006]. Most of these studies compared volume expansion alone with the combination of volume expansion and furosemide. The postprocedural increase in serum creatinine was either not significantly different or actually more pronounced in the groups receiving furosemide [Dussol et al., 2006]. In addition, the incidence of contrast nephropathy, defined as an increase in serum creatinine of ≥ 0.5 mg/dL, was higher in the furosemide group [Solomon et al., 1994]. A recent meta-analysis by Kelly et al., in which [Dobrowolski, Sadowski, 2005] randomized trials were reviewed, revealed that furosemide, mannitol, and the combination of furosemide, dopamine, and mannitol increased the risk of contrast nephropathy [Kelly et al., 2008]. A recent meta-analysis by Ho and Power [2010] also concluded that preventive furosemide administration does not improve the risk of RRT or mortality. On the basis of these results, the recent KDIGO guidelines recommended not using furosemide to prevent AKI (grade 1B) [Kellums et al., 2013] KDIGO guidelines declare that diuretics should not be used to treat AKI, except for the management of volume overload (grade 2C).

6.6.3.**Aminophylline.** The use of aminophylline for renal protection from acute kidney injury (AKI) is not novel. The efficacy of aminophylline for renal protection has been reported in patients receiving chemotherapy [Benoehr et al., 2005] and contrast-induced AKI [Dai et al., 2012], in animal models of kidney transplantation (20), and in the vasomotor nephropathy of very pre-term newborns [Catarelli et al., 2006]. However, its use in critically ill infants and children is not well described. Bell reported a small case series of 10 critically ill children who had a significant increase in urine output with theophylline administration [Bell et al., 1998]. However, in that report, there was no report of BUN or creatinine concentrations, and the concomitant use of low dose dopamine confounded the interpretation and the general applicability of the results. Intravenous infusion of theophylline, given to severely asphyxiated neonates within the first hour of birth, was associated with improved fluid balance, creatinine clearance, and reduced SCr levels and had no effects on neurological and respiratory complications [Jenik et al., 2008]. In another small retrospective case series, the administration of aminophylline to five neonates appeared to be associated with an increase in urine output; however, the lack of a bladder catheter complicated interpretation of the study results [Ng et al., 2005]. Lynch reported a retrospective case series of 13 neonates with non-oliguric AKI and described an improvement in renal function indices with aminophylline [Lynch et al., 2008]. However, in that publication, urine outputs were not reported, and many of the subjects were receiving concomitant caffeine, which shares similar properties of aminophylline. In a relatively recent retrospective study of nine children with AKI, aminophylline use resulted in improved urine flow rates, stable creatinine concentrations, and a reduced requirement for dialysis [Olowu, Adefehinti, 2012]. Although each of these studies supports a beneficial effect of aminophylline in renal injury, all have significant limitations. The purported renal benefits of aminophylline have been attributed to two mechanisms: adenosine receptor blockade at low dosage and type IV phosphodiesterase inhibition at high levels. Adenosine is the putative mediator of tubuloglomerular feedback [Li et al., 2012]. When the tubule is exposed to increased solute, energy depletion occurs, and adenosine is released. The released adenosine triggers preglomerular vasoconstriction thereby limiting solute flow and, in theory, restoring energy balance. In addition to adenosine receptor blockade, aminophylline-induced phosphodiesterase inhibition may prevent the hydrolysis of cAMP, which is important in the mediation of renal blood flow as it promotes renal vasodilatation [Thomas, Carcillo; 2013]. Both of these mechanisms likely contribute to the improved renal blood flow attributed to aminophylline. Current national guidelines only suggest that a single dose of theophylline may be administered to neonates with severe perinatal asphyxia at risk for AKI [KDIGO clinical practice guideline, 2012]. Recent studies show that aminophylline therapy may be associated with significantly improved renal excretory function and may augment urine output in children who experience oliguric acute kidney injury after CPB assisted surgery ICU [Axelrod et al., 2014].

6.7. Oxidative and inflammatory homeostasis.

The kidney has derangements in oxygen homeostasis during AKI. Although prospective study of CPB patients demonstrated that anemia is independently associated with AKI, the risks of increased volume and blood viscosity must be balanced against the presumed benefit of increased oxygen-carrying capacity. Studies of N-acetylcysteine and dexamethasone therapies to limit oxidative and inflammatory damage in AKI after CPB showed conflicting results [Rosner, Okusa, 2006]. The use of nephrotoxins such as aminoglycoside antimicrobials, nonsteroidal anti-inflammatory drugs, radiocontrast media, antifungal agents, and immunosuppressive drugs are associated with high rates of AKI and must be diligently constrained [Patzer, 2008].

6.8. Renal replacement therapy.

The selection of renal replacement modality will often reflect the experience and expertise of the individual center, rather than an objective criteria in the individual patient. Modality choice is also determined by a variety of factors, including provider preference, available institutional resources, dialytic goals and the specific advantages or disadvantages of each modality. As noted below, each modality of acute RRT can be successfully provided to pediatric patients of all sizes. Each program should evaluate which modality is provided most optimally and feasibly in its particular setting.

Selection of RRT modality. Specific indications for RRT typically include the need for ultrafiltration (i.e. fluid removal), either for symptomatic volume overload, or to make space for nutrition, medications, and blood product support and/or solute removal (i.e. urea, potassium), either for uremia or for removal of a dialyzable toxin. The rapid removal of solute (urea) and correction of electrolyte abnormalities (particularly elevated levels of potassium) are of extreme importance in the setting of AKI. While peritoneal dialysis (PD), intermittent hemodialysis (IHD) and continuous RRT (CRRT) can rapidly correct hyperkalemia and uremia, IHD and CRRT provide greater clearance of higher molecular weight solutes than PD. The rapidity of solute generation and its particular urgency for removal, as in tumor lysis syndrome, inborn errors of metabolism, hyperammonemia, symptomatic hyperkalemia, or ingestion of dialyzable toxins, require IHD or CRRT rather than PD, whereas mild uremia can be treated with any of the modalities. Mild volume overload can be treated with any modality. For example, a hemodynamically unstable patient with overwhelming sepsis, fluid overload, respiratory compromise, vasopressor requirements and renal involvement may necessitate initiation of CRRT for close fluid status control, whereas a postoperative cardiac patient with minimal fluid overload and hemodynamic instability may be better served by PD.

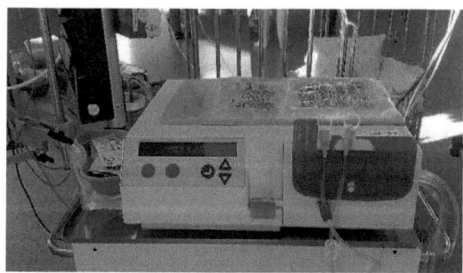

Fig. 1.   Automated cycling PD device (Baxter).

6.8.1.**Intracorporeal techniques**. From a technical aspect, PD can be relatively quickly and safely obtained, even in hemodynamically unstable patients and those with a coagulopathy. PD is superior in its requirement for less clinical expertise, fewer equipment resources, and cost. Given their small size and associated low blood volume,

PD may provide the least technically challenging option for infants and small children. Access in the form of classically surgically placed Tenckhoff catheters, or short-term PD or adapted PD catheters placed at the bedside percutaneously in patients unable to tolerate surgical placement, allow the rapid institution of therapy. PD has limitations for certain populations. Those with pulmonary compromise may have a worsening of their symptoms due to increased abdominal dialysate volumes, thereby preventing full diaphragmatic excursion. Patients with ventriculoperitoneal shunts or prune belly syndrome have been successfully dialyzed with PD but do present increased potential complications. Finally, patients that have undergone abdominal surgery may not be amenable to utilizing this therapy, and, in patients with diaphragmatic defects, the use of PD is contraindicated. The process of PD itself can cause significant losses in immunoglobulins, increasing the risk of infections in these patients. Peritonitis can lead to further increased dialysate protein loss, nutritional compromise, loss of ultrafiltration capacity, and permanent damage to the peritoneal membrane. Mechanical complications associated with PD include leaks, hernias and catheter obstruction. Dialysate leakage may occur around the catheter or into the pleural space, resulting in hydrothorax. Drainage problems seen with PD are typically caused from catheter malfunctions in the form of omentum and fibrin clot obstructions. The potential for complications from infections must not be overlooked, and the clinician must vigilant to the possibility of peritonitis, particularly fungal peuritonitis. Althogh an automated cycler provides a precise measurement of ultrafiltration, manual exchanges are inexpensive and technically simple and can provide an efficient form of dialysis if an remain automated machine is not available or if the infant is so small that the starting exchange volume is below the minimum permitted by the cycler. However, warming of dialysate is difficult without the use of an automatic cycler. In the critical-care setting, warming of PD solution is often difficult and overlooked, yet it is an important component for maintaining hemodynamic stability and improving effective solute clearance. A PD nurse specialist can teach ICU nurses to perform manual exchanges quickly, which avoids the need for a specialized dialysis nurse to continuously remain at bedside. The dialysis prescription should be adjusted according to the patient's needs. Basic principles include the use of frequent, continuous exchanges, with low volumes of dialysate. Exchanges with volumes as low as 10 – 20 mL/kg body weight (300 – 600 mL/m2) not only help prevent dialysate leakage and respiratory complications from compression of the lungs, but also have been shown to provide adequate ultrafiltration rates in critically ill children [Golej et al., 2002]. Dwell

36

times as short as 20 minutes are effective in infants younger than 12 months, although short dwells carry a risk of sodium sieving [Alarabi et al., 1994].

6.8.2.**Extracorporeal techniques**. Recent advances in technology and safety of RRT have changed the practice of pediatric nephrologists significantly in the last three decades. In 1990 only 41% offered extracorporeal RRT modalities to infants younger than 1 month. Technological advances aimed at providing accurate ultrafiltration with volumetric control incorporated into CRRT equipment, and disposable lines, circuits, and dialyzers sized for the entire pediatric weight spectrum have made CRRT safer and feasible for children of all ages and sizes [Symons et al., 2003; 2007].

6.8.2.1. **IHD (Intermittent hemodialysis).** IHD requires technical expertise on the part of the physician, nurse and technician for optimal support for the wide range of pediatric patients, and, typically, it is available in larger secondary and tertiary care hospitals. Vascular access is essential and most important component contributing to the satisfactory provision of this therapy. Shortness and large diameter of the cannulas were

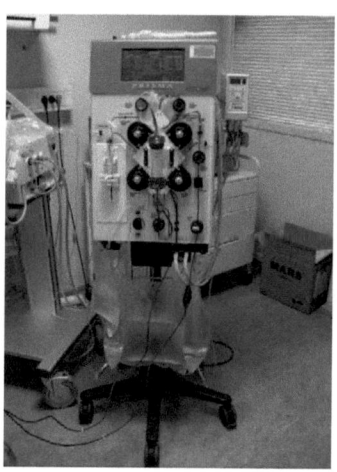

Fig. 2. Prismaflex CRRT machine

critical to achieve a good blood flow while avoiding unnecessary pressure loss. Flexibility without any reduction of the inner lumen of the cannula and good clinical tolerance were two other important features of the vascular access. Several vascular access routes were been utilized in infants in the early 1980s, including umbilical vessels and brachial artery or femoral artery cannulation (with surgical isolation of the artery). Flexible Teflon cannulas (18–20 gauge) that were 20–25 mm long were generally employed. Mean arterial pressure in the newborn generally ranged from 35 to 50 mmHg, resulting in blood flows

ranging from 15 to 40 ml/min [11]. Cannulation of the brachial or femoral artery in infants led in some cases to distal hypoperfusion of the arm and had to be replaced. The jugular or subclavian veins were the most common route for venous return, while femoral veins were avoided if at all possible. In neonates the use of umbilical veins is an important consideration for vascular access. Utilization of neck veins, although limited by anatomy, may be preferable, especially in infants weighing less than 5 kg. Such access may allow for less recirculation and avoid the potential high venous return pressures often associated with groin lines in patients with high intra-abdominal pressures. While difficult in the smallest infants, it is possible. A wide variety of temporary vascular catheters are available for the pediatric population. Placement of temporary or permanent vascular catheters for IHD can result in blood vessel stenosis or thrombosis, along with air emboli or hemorrhage. Depending on location or degree of difficulty involved in the placement of short-term or permanent vascular catheters, future access needs may be compromised. This issue becomes of great importance for patients requiring long term access that progress from acute to chronic kidney injury. If possible, subclavian catheter placement should be avoided altogether, due to the very high incidence of stenosis at the puncture site, which may render the formation of a fistula impossible in the future. IHD can be utilized without anticoagulation and does not require the extra central line placement often needed.

6.8.2.1.2. **CRRT (Continous renal replacement therapy).** As with IHD, adequate vascular access is required for CRRT. This technical aspect is the most important consideration contributing to the effectiveness of the therapy. Depending on the type of anticoagulation used, an additional central line may be required, as with regional citrate anticoagulation. Historically, arteriovenous circuits were utilized; however, these have given way to commercially available venovenous therapies, which are pump driven and provide more predictable blood flow and, therefore, solute and ultrafiltration rates. Despite the availability of smaller circuits in some jurisdictions, the large extracorporeal volume required for CRRT and IHD (particularly in neonates) is a distinct disadvantage, necessitating blood priming in patients weighing less than 10 kg. In these settings, extracorporeal blood volume exceeds 10% of the patient's blood volume. This exposes the patient to obvious risks associated with blood products and hemodynamic instability related to the flow of blood out of the body. Patients with multiple organ failure and hemodynamic instability may not tolerate the rapid circulation of blood through a CRRT circuit, regardless of the patient's size [Strazdins et al., 2004]. Additionally, depending on the types of hemofilters utilized, hemodynamic instability may be observed with CRRT due to bradykinin reactions, activation of complement-coagulation cascade-monocytes, neutrophil degranulation and/or the release of reactive oxygen species [Brophy et al., 2001]. Some of the more significant technical disadvantages of CRRT include the requirement for continuous anticoagulation [Brophy et al., 2005] and the clotting of circuits. While many easy anticoagulation protocols are available, anticoagulation comes with its own set of complications. The predictability and efficiency of ultrafiltration (UF) and solute removal make CRRT ideally suited for the provision of RRT in hemodynamically unstable patients. A particular advantage afforded by CRRT (and IHD) is the ability for ultrafiltration to be separated from solute removal, which allows more flexibility for prescriptions to be tailored to the patient's needs. Minimal requirements for fluid restriction, due to predictable and continual fluid removal while CRRT is being performed, allow improved and adequate nutritional delivery. The need for supplemental protein (as high as 3–4 gm/kg per day) during CRRT must not be underestimated when this therapy is being used, as the sieving coefficients of most aminoacids are close to 1, and, therefore, clearance is quite high and can result in a nutritional deficit [Maxvold et al., 2000]. In the setting of AKI, CRRT can rapidly and predictably restore homeostasis. Indeed, CRRT provides superior uremia control compared to PD [Fleming et al., 1995] or even intermittent daily hemodialysis. Alteration of dialysate or filter replacement fluid is possible and can allow the clinician to control electrolyte levels within a desired target range; this is particularly important in the setting of increased intracranial pressure, when higher sodium levels may be required or when hyperosmolar states need to be corrected [McBryde et al., 2005]. Of course, due to potential compounding errors, caution needs to be exercised when these alterations are being made, and they should be done under careful guidance of the clinician and pharmacist [Barletta et al., 2006]. CRRT during AKI may have the additional benefit of restoring immuno-homeostasis via removal of both proinflammatory and anti-inflammatory molecules [Ronco et al., 2004]. This remains an area of active ongoing research. New possibilities for newborns and infants,

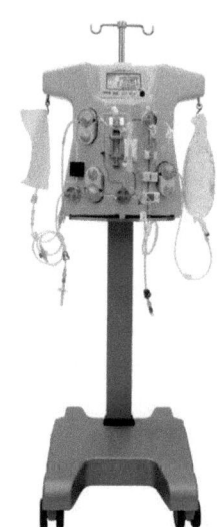

Fig. 3. CARPEDIEM CRRT machine with dimensions: 44 (L) × 43 (H) ×23 (W) cm, weighs 13 kg.
With permission of Bellco

requiring RRT arise after introduction of miniaturized RRT machine CARPEDIEM with low priming volume of the circuit (<30mL), miniaturized roller pumps, and accurate ultrafiltration control via calibrated scales with a precision of 1g [Ronco et al.,2014]. Authors describe the successful use of machine for a 2,9-kg neonate with hemorrhagic shock, multiple organ dysfunction, and severe fluid overload for more than 400 h was treated with the CARPEDIEM, using continuous venovenous hemofiltration, single-pass albumin dialysis, blood exchange, and plasma exchange. Other device, the NIDUS [Coulthard et al., 2014] is an HD circuit with a capability of treating babies weighing between 800 g and 8 kg. The extracorporeal circuit volume < 10ml, and thus even in the smallest of babies, no blood prime is required. The most innovative feature of the NIDUS is the uncoupling of blood flow through the dialyser from the baby's blood flow. A prescribed volume of blood is removed from the patient and then passes twice through a high flux polysulfone 0,045 m^2 hollow-fibre haemofilter to allow dialysis and UF and is then returned to the baby; the cycle is repeated. This strategy also makes it possible to dialyse infants through a single-lumen catheter without excessive recirculation. The UF capability of the circuit is 0–60 ml/h, and UF accuracy matches that of the CARPEDIEM. Comparison of different RRT modalities are summarized in the Table 6.:

Table 6   **Advantages and disadvantages of various modalities of**
              renal replacement therapy for acute kidney injury

Variable	Peritoneal dialysis	Intermittent hemodialysis	CRRT
Continuous therapy	Yes	No	Yes
Hemodynamic stability	Yes	No	Yes
Fluid removal	Yes/no, variable	No	Yes
Toxin removal	Depends on toxin size	No	Yes
Complexity	No	Yes	Yes
Optimal nutrition	No	No	Yes
Anticoagulation	No	Intermittent	Yes
Vascular access	No	Yes	Yes
Recent abdominal surgery	No	Yes	Yes
Nursing support	Moderate	Low	High
Use in inborn metabolic errors	No	No	Yes
Cost	Low-Moderate	Moderate-High	High

6.8.3.**Outcome using different RRT modalities**. In the study made by Fleming et al., [1995] authors retrospectively compared PD (n=21) and CRRT (n=21) in 42 children following repair of congenital heart disease lesions. The common indications for RRT implementation included fluid overload, electrolyte abnormalities, provision of total parenteral nutrition (TPN), and oliguria. No standardized initiation criteria were utilized, and this varied significantly among patients. Additionally, nine patients in the CRRT group received arteriovenous CRRT. Most of the patients (90%) required vasopressor support. While there was no difference noted in terms of mortality rate between modalities (62% for both), CRRT was superior to PD for ultrafiltration, solute clearance and nutritional provision. From these data, the authors concluded that CRRT was superior to PD in this clinical setting. The conclusions of their study must be guarded, as patient care was not standardized in terms of modality initiation criterion. Also, the patient group was rather homogeneous, making generalizability difficult, and no apparent survival benefit was noted with improved solute and ultrafiltration in the CRRT group. Bunchman et al., [2001] reviewed survival outcome in 226 pediatric patients receiving various forms of RRT, including PD, IHD and CRRT, over a 7-year period from 1992–1998. Patients were treated with CRRT (n=106), IHD (n=61) or PD (n=59). Factors influencing patient survival included: (1) low blood pressure (BP) at the initiation of RRT (33% survival, low BP; 61%, normal BP; 100%, high BP; P<0.05); (2) vasopressor use anytime during RRT (35% survival on vasopressors; 89% survival not requiring pressors; P<0.01); (3) diagnosis (improved outcome in those with primary renal failure compared to those with secondary renal failure; P<0.05); (4) RRT modality (40% survival, CRRT; 49% survival, PD; 81% survival, IHD; P<0.01 IHD vs PD or CRRT), and (5) vasopressor support was significantly higher in children on CRRT (74%) and PD (81%) vs IHD (33%) (P<0.05 IHD vs CRRT or PD). The authors concluded that hemodynamic support (sicker patients) with vasopressors imparted a greater prediction of mortality, rather than RRT modality, and that survival of children, as of adults, is best predicted by the underlying diagnosis and hemodynamic stability. Interestingly, modality choice was determined, in part, by patient status. That is, patients with greater hemodynamic instability were preferentially treated with PD or CRRT, and many of these patients required vasopressor support.

6.8.4.**Summary of RRT:** The indications for RRT in pediatric patients with AKI have changed over the years, and the present trend is towards a wider spectrum of applications, including the prevention of fluid accumulation and MODS [Bailey et al., 2007]. At the present time, PD is the RRT treatment of choice in neonates, unless specific contraindications are present (i.e., peritonitis, abdominal masses, or bleeding). However, in PD, UF and solute clearance occur rather slowly and efficiency is suboptimal Extracorporeal dialysis in children can be managed with a variety of modalities, including intermittent HD, and continuous hemofiltration or hemodiafiltration. The choice of dialysis modality to be used is influenced by several factors, including the goals of the dialysis, the unique advantages and disadvantages of each modality, and institutional resources. Intermittent dialysis may not be well tolerated in infants because of rapid rate of fluid removal and of osmotic shifts secondary to sudden solute clearance: this condition is particularly evident in hemodynamically unstable, critically ill pediatric patients [Flynn et al., 2002]. A specific indication to intermittent dialysis is the presence of severe hyperammonemia refractory to medical therapy [Picca et al., 2001]. Critically ill children, however, are generally treated by CRRT, which allows for slow fluid removal, solute re-equilibration and, probably, the removal of pro-inflammatory mediators. To date, however, outcomes of critically ill children with AKI are poor, and a strategy for improvement is urgently needed. In this scenario, new technological advances, such as miniaturized circuits and membranes and accurate CRRT machines, as well as effective prescription schedules provide promise to the clinician for improving the quality of treatment.

6.9. Nutritional Support.

Patients who develop AKI, especially in the intensive care unit (ICU), are at risk of protein–energy malnutrition, which is a major negative prognostic factor in this clinical condition. Despite the lack of evidence from controlled trials of its effect on outcome, nutritional support by the enteral (preferentially) and/or parenteral route appears clinically indicated in most cases of ICU-acquired AKI, independently of the actual nutritional status of the patient, in order to prevent deterioration in the nutritional state with all its known complications. Extrapolating from data in other conditions, it seems intrinsically unlikely that starvation of a catabolic patient is more beneficial than appropriate nutritional support by an expert team with the skills to avoid the potential complications of the enteral and parenteral nutrition methodologies. The primary goals of nutritional support in AKI, which represents a well-known inflammatory and prooxidative condition, are the same as those for other critically ill patients with normal renal function, i.e. to ensure the delivery of adequate nutrition, to prevent protein–energy wasting with its attendant metabolic complications, to promote wound healing and tissue repair, to support immune system function, to accelerate recovery and to reduce mortality. Patients with AKI on RRT should receive a basic intake of at least 1,5 g/kg/day of protein with an additional 0,2 g/kg/day to compensate for amino acid/protein loss during RRT, especially when daily treatments and/or high efficiency modalities are used. Energy intake should consist of no more than 30 kcal non-protein calories or $1,3 \times$ BEE (Basal Energy Expenditure) calculated by the Harris–Benedict equation, with ~30–35% from lipid, as lipid emulsions. For nutritional support, the enteral route is preferred, although it often needs to be supplemented through the parenteral route in order to meet nutritional requirements. In the past, nutrition intervention was often postponed in patients with renal insufficiency to delay dialysis [Star, 1998], because nutrition support may contribute to azotemia, fluid overload, and electrolyte disturbances. Because of the catabolic nature of the illness associated with kidney injury, it is now recognized that standard recommendations for energy and protein are appropriate for ICU patients with AKI [McClave et al., 2009]. Most of the available pediatric data for nutritional risk in renal disease come from studies focusing on patients with CKD. Pediatric patients on hemodialysis with severe growth failure have a 3-fold increase in mortality compared with the same age cohorts [Wong et al., 2000]. Supplemental parenteral nutrition during CRRT has been successfully used to reverse weight loss and to promote weight gain for pediatric hemodialysis patients [Orellana et al., 2005]. Enteral nutrition is safe in most adult patients with AKI; moreover, those on renal replacement therapy may require higher protein as intravenous infusions to compensate for protein losses in the dialysate [Flaccadori et al., 2004]. Nutritional recommendations for pediatric AKI are limited to patients receiving renal replacement therapy. As generally observed in the critically ill [Kreymann et al., 2006], also in patients with AKI energy expenditure seems to depend more on the severity of the underlying disease, pre-existing nutritional status and acute/chronic comorbidities, than on the presence of the syndrome itself [Toygo et al., 2000, Faisy et al., 2003]. In a recent survey of the nutritional management of 195 children with AKI on CRRT, the maximal calorie prescription in the course of treatment averaged 53, 31, and 21 kcal/kg/day, and that for protein intake 2,4; 1,9; and 1,3 g/kg/day in children aged <1 year, 1 to 13 years, and >13 years, respectively [Zapitelli et al., 2008]. Although not validated by outcome studies, these figures provide an orientation for the macronutrient supply typically achieved in and tolerated by children with AKI receiving CRRT. Energy expenditure measured by indirect calorimetry rarely exceeds 1,3 times the basal energy expenditure (BEE) calculated by the Harris–Benedict equation, corresponding to 20–25 non-protein kcal/kg/day. The optimal protein intake of AKI patients is ill defined: as protein catabolic rate (PCR) in this clinical condition varies from 1,4 to 1,8 g/kg/day [Btaiche et al., 2008], an intake of at least 0,25 g of nitrogen/day is required to achieve less negative or nearly positive nitrogen balance. Evidence from RCTs concerning advantages of very high protein intakes in critically ill patients with AKI is lacking. With 2,5 g/kg/day of protein and 35 kcal/kg/day of energy, only one-third of patients achieved a positive nitrogen balance [45]; in a cross-over study on AKI patients receiving an isocaloric regimen—in most cases through EN—nitrogen balance was positively related to protein intake, with a positive nitrogen balance being more likely to be obtained with intakes >2 g/kg/day (0,3 g nitrogen/kg/day) [Scheinkestel et al., 2003]. However, in many patients with AKI, hypercatabolism cannot simply be overcome by increasing protein or amino acid intake much above 0,25– 0,3 g nitrogen/kg/day, even when energy intake is optimal. It is likely that above this level of nitrogen intake any further increase contributes nothing to protein synthesis, simply increasing urea production. Both EEA and NEAA are recommended in AKI, since a higher provision of EEA only does not appear to be advantageous [12,13]. No data are currently available for other specific amino acids, e.g. glutamine. Nutritional support is able to significantly increase amino acid levels in AKI patients [Berg et al., 2007]. Protein and amino acid losses through the extracorporeal circulation of RRT can be

44

quantified as ~0,2 g amino acids/l of ultrafiltrate (up to 10–15 g amino acids per day), and 5–10 g/day of protein [Maxyold et al., 2000]; in order to compensate for these losses, especially when highflux filters and/or highly efficient modalities (such as CRRT or SLED (Sustained low efficiency dialysis) are used, the protein intake should be increased by ~0,2 g/kg/day. For relatively non-catabolic AKI patients with the milder nonoliguric forms of the syndrome not needing RRT and who are likely to regain renal function in a few days (drug toxicity, contrast nephropathy, etc.), lower protein intakes (up to 0,8 g/kg/day) will suffice for short periods of time, combined with adequate calorie intakes (30 kcal/kg/day) [Cano et al., 2009]. The optimal energy to nitrogen ratio has not been clearly defined in patients with AKI. In an observational study of patients on CRRT, less negative or weakly positive nitrogen balance values were predicted by linear regression analysis models when protein intakes of 1,5 g/kg BW/day were provided in parallel with non-protein energy intakes of ~25 kcal/kg BW/day; simply increasing the calorie to nitrogen ratio in this study was not invariably associated with better nitrogen balance [Macias et al., 1996]. With a protein intake of 1,5 g/kg/day, an increase in energy provision up to 40 kcal/g/day did not improve nitrogen balance compared with lower energy intakes (30 kcal/kg/day); instead, more severe metabolic complications (hypertriglyceridaemia, hyperglycaemia) ensued. Lipids should represent ~30–35% of total nonprotein energy supply [Cano et al., 2009]. In the case of parenteral nutrition, this can be obtained by giving the patient 0,8–1,2 g/kg/day of lipid from 10 to 30% lipid emulsions or as a part of the commercially available three-in-one total nutrient admixtures. Lipids should be infused over 18–24 h, and serum tryglycerides should be monitored, stopping lipid administration when tryglycerides exceed 400 mg/dl. Even though the use of parenteral MCT may result theoretically in lower serum triglyceride levels because of faster oxidation rate, pharmacokinetic studies failed to show any clear advantages, in terms of plasma clearance of trygliceride, of the mixed MCT/LCT lipid formulas compared with LCT only emulsions [Druml et al., 1992]. Lipid losses through the filters do not occur during haemodialysis or haemofiltration.

6.9.1.**Trace elements, vitamins and electrolytes**. Levels of trace elements (essential micronutrients with regulatory, immunologic and antioxidant functions) can be lower than normal in AKI [Fiaccadori et al., 2005]. This can be due to many factors: acute phase reaction/critical illness, leading to variable protein binding, redistribution of elements between plasma and tissues, acute losses of biological fluids, dilution, varying concentrations of trace elements in dialysis/haemofiltration fluids, effects of enteral or parenteral nutrition fluid, analytical problems, etc. Moreover, RRT fluids (dialysis fluid or sterile solutions for fluid replacement in the case of haemofiltration) may have variable content of trace elements, at concentrations often difficult to detect; finally, the effects of RRT on the removal of mainly protein-bound trace elements are far from being clearly defined. Data from *in vitro* studies indicate that selenium, chromium, copper and zinc can be removed from plasma by convective/diffusive RRT's [Nakamura et al., 2004]. In the clinical setting, CVVH is associated with reduced plasma selenium and zinc but high chromium levels; there was a little loss of the former two elements in the ultrafiltrate, whereas considerable losses of chromium and copper were observed [Story et al., 1999]. Zinc was detected in effluent fluid in CVVHDF, but zinc balance was nonetheless positive, owing to the zinc content of PN and replacement fluid solutions, and its presence as a contaminant of the anticoagulant solution (trisodium citrate). These sources when combined exceeded the losses due to CRRT. In contrast, the association of convection and diffusion in CVVHDF was associated with selenium losses, regardless of the buffer solution used, resulting in a daily negative balance equivalent to twice the daily intake from standard formula parenteral nutrition fluids [Metnitz et al., 2000]. Thus, patients with AKI are at risk of trace element depletion; however, the precise requirements have not been clearly defined. In ICU patients with AKI, plasma levels of water-soluble vitamins, such as vitamin C, thiamine and folic acid, may be lower than normal, due mainly to the losses occurring through the extracorporeal circuit: in CVVH vitamin C losses can reach up to 600 μmol/day, i.e. 100 mg/day, and folate losses up to 600 nmol/day [Story et al., 1999; Berger et al., 2004]; in CVVHDF thiamine losses may amount more than 1,5 times the daily provision of the vitamin from standard total parenteral nutrition solutions. While in experimental AKI, plasma retinol levels are increased, in clinical conditions serum levels of vitamin A and vitamin E can be decreased [Cano et al., 2009; Druml 2001]; the risk of hypervitaminosis A and vitamin A-related toxicity seems to be increased in pediatric patients with AKI receiving artificial nutrition, especially parenteral nutrition . The activation of vitamin D3 is impaired in AKI [Cano et al., 2009]. Recommended vitamin C administration in patients with AKI is 50–100 mg/day; higher intakes (up to 150–200 mg) may be needed when continuous modalities of RRT are used. No supplementation of fat-soluble vitamins is usually necessary in AKI. Derangements in fluid, electrolyte and acid–base equilibrium, such as hypo- and hypernatraemia, hyperkalaemia, hyperphosphataemia, metabolic acidosis, etc.,

46

commonly occur in critically ill patients with AKI. Intensive (daily) RRT can readily correct these abnormalities by appropriate regulation of the composition of haemodialysis/haemofiltration fluids and of the intensity of RRT. The highly efficient modalities of RRT often induce hypophosphataemia and hypomagnesaemia, abnormalities that that can be prevented by adequate electrolyte supplementation.

6.9.2.**Effects of nutritional support on patient outcome in AKI**. Due to the heterogeneity/complexity of the syndrome, and to major methodological flaws in the available studies, the advantages of nutritional support in AKI remain controversial, especially in highly catabolic patients, and nor are there clear indications about the optimal timing of artificial nutrition. Studies published during the 1980s analysed the effect of parenteral nutrition on mortality, but they are largely underpowered. In three prospective studies [Feinstein et al., 1981; 1983, Mirtallo et al., 1982] no survival advantage was demonstrated. However, such studies were methodologically flawed also by due to suboptimal selection of patients, population heterogeneity, lack of stratification for severity of illness, nutritional status, RRT dose received, use of historical controls, quantitative and qualitative inadequacy of caloric and nitrogen intake, etc. In a prospective trial assessing calorie and protein needs of critically ill anuric patients requiring CRRT, nitrogen balance was positively related to protein intake and more likely to be attained with protein intakes of >2 g/kg/day [Scheinkestel et al., 2003]. Similar data were obtained in a group of patients with milder forms of nonoliguric AKI [Winchester et al., 1989]. Negative nitrogen balance has been associated with worse ICU and hospital outcomes in AKI patients receiving mixed nutritional support (enteral plus parenteral) [Scheinkestel et al., 2003]; in the same study, the use of the enteral route had a statistically significant advantage in terms of outcome. Enteral nutrition was also associated with a positive outcome in a large observational cohort of AKI patients in the ICU [Metnitz et al., 2002]. There is sparse and indirect evidence suggesting that amino acids might favour the recovery of renal function. Intravenously or enterally administered amino acids increase renal plasma flow and glomerular filtration rate in animals and in normal subjects [Winchester et al., 1989], and GFR can improve moderately following an amino acid load in chronic renal failure. However, the information available on the possible beneficial effects of amino acids in patients with AKI is scarce. In one experimental study, enteral nutrition (EN) was superior to parenteral in this respect [Mouser et al., 1997]. A positive effect of a high amino acid parenteral regimen on renal function in terms of diuresis preservation and water balance has been suggested recently in patients with nonoliguric forms of AKI [Singer, 2007].

6.9.3.**Indications for nutritional support and route of feeding in AKI**. The indications for nutritional support in AKI are not quite different from those established for the other critically ill patients [Kreymann et al., 2006]. In the same way, also in this clinical setting the route of feeding depends more on gastrointestinal tract (GI) function than on the presence of the syndrome itself. Thus, in AKI the enteral route should be the first choice for nutritional support if the GI tract is functioning, while parenteral nutrition should be reserved when GI tract cannot be used, or when EN appears inadequate to reach nutrient intake goals [Fiaccadori et al., 2004]. Renal failure can impair gastrointestinal motility. Apart from AKI itself, other factors commonly present in critically ill patients are known to impair GI function, e.g. medications such as sedatives, opiates or catecholamines; hyperglycaemia; electrolyte disorders; mechanical ventilation, etc. Finally, AKI is a well-defined risk factor for upper-gastrointestinal bleeding [Fiaccadori et al., 2001]; it is uncertain whether enteral nutrition has any protective effects on this risk. Enteral nutrition is safe and effective in AKI, even though data are scanty. No evidence was found that AKI is associated with a consistent increase of gastrointestinal, mechanical or metabolic complications during enteral nutrition in an observational study on 182 patients with AKI, receiving either a standard formula or a disease-specific formula for patients with renal failure on haemodialysis [Fiaccadori et al., 2001]. High gastric residual volumes were the most frequent side effect. Underdelivery of targeted energy intakes due to enteral nutrition-related complications was rarely observed. Although standard enteral formulae are adequate for the majority of critically ill patients with AKI, the use of disease-specific (renal) formulae designed for patients with chronic renal failure may afford some advantage, due to their high energy (2 kcal/ml) and protein content (70 g/l) and low electrolyte levels; however, even with the most suitable disease-specific enteral formulae, parenteral supplementation of amino acids is likely to be required in order to meet the targeted nitrogen requirement. In patients with AKI in the ICU, the combination of enteral and parenteral feeding allows successful nutritional support in most cases [Scheinstel et al., 2003]: thus, the two routes of nutritional support are to be considered complementary and not mutually exclusive [Cano et al., 2006]. Standard formulae for parenteral nutrition (amino acids solutions and commercial three-in-one nutrient admixtures) containing both essential and non-essential are to be preferred in AKI on RRT. In some patients, three-in-one nutrient admixtures without electrolytes (i.e. without

48

sodium, potassium, etc.) are now commercially available, and can be used with caution and careful monitoring or customized according to patient needs. Whether immune enhancing diets should be given to AKI patients remains unsettled. For short time periods, peripheral PN can be used in AKI patients, according to fluid restriction needs and calorie/protein goals. Due to the need of fluid restriction and the high osmolarity of more concentrated commercial three-in-one admixtures, parenteral nutrition in AKI patients, especially those in the ICU, must be infused in a central vein.

7. Outcome of AKI.

It has been thought that AKI due to hypoxic/ischemic and nephrotoxic insults were reversible, with a return of renal function to normal. However, recent studies have demonstrated that hypoxic/ischemic and nephrotoxic insults can lead to physiologic and morphologic alterations in the kidney that may lead to kidney disease at a later time [Zager, 1996]. Since nephrogenesis is not complete until approximately 34 weeks gestation, AKI during this interval might lead to a decreased number of nephrons, and, indeed studies have suggested that AKI during nephrogenesis results in decreased numbers of nephrons and subsequent glomerulomegaly [Rodriguez et al., 2005]. Premature neonates provide an informative pediatric population for study since they can be exposed to numerous nephrotoxic insults (e.g. sepsis, nephrotoxic medications) before nephrogenesis is complete White et al. [2009] recently performed a meta-analysis of studies examining low birth weight infants and CKD development later in life. After reviewing 1,600 studies, they were able to include 32 papers comprising 17 case-control or cohort studies (46,249 patients) and 1 genetic record linkage study. Low birth weight, defined as birth weight between 1,500 and 2,500 g, imparted a 70% risk of developing CKD later in life (HR: 1,73, 95% CI: 1.44–2.08) and an 80% greater risk of developing albuminuria later in life (HR: 1,81; 95% CI: 1,19–2,77) compared to normal birth weight infants. AKI in the full-term neonate is also associated with later kidney disease [Polito et al., 1998]. Studies on older children have also shown that AKI leads to CKD in a higher percentage of children than was previously appreciated [Askenazi et al., 2006]. In a prospective study of renal insufficiency in children undergoing bone marrow transplantation, the incidence of acute renal insufficiency was high and was predictive of chronic renal insufficiency. Of those who survived, 11% developed CKD, and AKI was the sole predictor of CKD [Kist-van Holthe et al., 2002]. The short-term outcomes of children with AKI as a complication of critical illness are also well known. In a multicenter retrospective analysis of 2,106 pediatric ICU admissions, AKI was independently associated with longer ICU stay and mechanical ventilation [Alkandari et al., 2011]. A recent large retrospective study of 3,396 admissions to a single pediatric ICU illustrated that those who presented with AKI on admission had a 32% mortality rate and those who developed AKI at any time during the ICU stay had a 30% mortality rate [Shneider et al., 2010]. Remarkably, this persistently high mortality rate of 30–40% in critically ill children with AKI has been consistently demonstrated in several very recent studies [Duzova et al., 2010].

Thus, notwithstanding advances in pediatric renal and critical care, severe AKI requiring renal replacement therapy in children is still associated with a mortality rate of 30–50%, and this has not changed appreciably over the past two decades. This may reflect, in part, the fact that those with severe AKI also have increasing severity of their primary illness, so that an improvement in survival rates is not readily apparent despite renal replacement therapy. This notion is supported by a multicenter retrospective analysis of 344 children requiring continuous renal replacement therapy, in whom the overall mortality rate was 42% (Symons et al., 2007). However, there was significantly better survival in patients with less severity of their primary illness, including drug intoxication (100%), primary renal disease (84%), and tumor lysis syndrome (83%). Despite dialysis, survival was lowest in the sickest children with liver disease (43%), pulmonary disease (45%), and bone marrow transplant (45%).

 The previous assumption that patients who survived an episode of AKI would recover kidney function has been challenged. A recent meta-analysis of 13 published cohort studies showed that adults with AKI are at a 9-fold higher risk of developing CKD, and a 3-fold increased risk of developing ESRD, when compared to patients without AKI [Coca et al., 2012]. Similar evidence is accumulating in the pediatric population [Garg et al., 2003]. In a prospective study of children who developed AKI and were followed up for 3–5 years, 60% developed evidence for CKD (proteinuria, decreased GFR, hypertension), 9% developed ESRD, and 20% died (Askenazi et al. 2006). A shorter 1–3 year follow up of 126 critically ill children who suffered an episode of AKI [Mammen et al., 2012] showed that 10% developed CKD (eGFR < 60 ml/min per 1,73 m^2 or albuminuria), but 47% showed evidence of CKD risk (eGFR 60–90 ml/min per 1,73 m^2 or hypertension). However, several unknowns remain. Can clinical risk factors (e.g. etiology and severity of AKI, pre-existing CKD, other co-morbid factors) determine the risk of CKD after AKI? Can novel biomarkers predict this risk? Can early interventions prevent progression of CKD? Ongoing long-term follow up studies in both children and adults [Go et al., 2010] are expected to clarify some of these questions, but clearly a lot more work is needed to strengthen the emerging recommendation that children with AKI require long-term evaluation for CKD. Future studies should also incorporate lessons learned from contemporary basic science studies that have unveiled the mechanisms leading to vascular rarefaction and progressive interstitial fibrosis after AKI [Basile et al., 2011], and the role of novel regulatory proteins such as neutrophil gelatinase-associated lipocalin and kidney injury molecule-1 as pathogenic factors as well as early biomarkers for the AKI-

51

to-CKD transition. In the recent study [Cooper et al., 2014] it has been shown that a novel biomarker uL-FABP remain elevated even 5 years after the CPB associated AKI. Thus, children with a history of AKI from any cause need long-term follow-up.

8.CONCLUSION

The management of AKI in pediatrics is complex and challenging. Our understanding and ability to detect renal distress are in their infancy. Biomarkers may improve our management if early detection actually affects outcomes. To date, therapy of AKI revolves around optimizing renal perfusion pressure and oxygenation through a combination of judicious fluid prescription, inotropy, and RRT while attending to proper nutrition and avoidance of additional nephrotoxins. However, pediatric intensivists have limited consensus or best-practice parameters to follow, as little prospective evidence is available. Kidney injury is likely incremental, more temporally proximal than fluid overload and anuric failure, and likely causes more significant distal harm than previously appreciated. The impact of AKI on critically ill children is significant and demands prospective study if we are to find effective therapies and improve outcomes.

References:

1. Abuelo JG: Normotensive ischemic acute renal failure. N Engl J Med 2007, 357:797-805.

2. Akcan-Arikan A., Zappitelli M., Loftis L.L, Washburn K.K, Jefferson L.S, Goldstein S.L (2007). Modified RIFLE criteria in critically ill children with acute kidney injury. Kidney Int;71:1028–1035.

3. Akech S., Gwer S., Idro R., Fegan G, Eziefula AC., Newton C.R.J., Levin M., Maitland K.(2006). Volume Expansion with Albumin Compared to Gelofusine in Children with Severe Malaria: Results of a Controlled Trial.PLoSClin Trials.;1(5): e21. Published online Sep 15, 2006.

4. Akech, S., Ledermann H., Maitland K. (2010). Choice of fluids for resuscitation in children with severe infection and shock: systematic review. BMJ; 341:c4416.

5. Alarabi AA, Petersson T, Danielson BG, Wikström B. Continuous peritoneal dialysis in children with acute renal failure. Adv Perit Dial 1994; 10:289–93.

6. Alkandari O, Eddington KA, Hyder A, Gauvin F, Ducruet T, Gottesman R, Phan V, Zappitelli M. Acute kidney injury is an independent risk factor for pediatric intensive care unit mortality, longer length of stay and prolonged mechanical ventilation in critically ill children: a two-center retrospective cohort study. Crit Care. 2011; 15(3):R146.

7. Andoni G., Zangrillo A., Cabrini L., Monti G., Turi S., Bignami E., Biondi-Zoccai G.L., Sheiban I. (2012). Continuous infusion versus bolus injection of furosemide in pediatric patients after cardiac surgery: A meta-analysis of randomized studies, SIGNA VITAE; 7(1):17-22.

8. Andreoli S.P. Acute renal failure. (2002). Curr Opin Pediatr ;14:183–188.

9. Andreoli S.P. (2009) Acute kidney injury in children. Pediatr Nephrol; 24:253–263.

10. Antonelli M., Levy M., Andrews P.J., Chastre J., Hudson L.D., Manthous C., Meduri G.U., Moreno R.P., Putensen C., Stewart T., Torres A. (2007). Hemodynamic monitoring in shock and implications for management: International Consensus Conference, Paris, France, 27–28 April 2006. Intensive Care Med; 33:575–590.

11. Arikan AA, Zappitelli M, Goldstein SL, Naipaul A, Jefferson LS, Loftis LL. Fluid overload is associated with impaired oxygenation and morbidity in critically ill children. Pediatr Crit Care Med 2012; 13:253-258.

12. Askenazi D.J., Feig D.I., Graham N.M., Hui-Stickle S., Goldstein S. (2006). 1-5 year longitudinal follow-up of pediatric patients after acute renal failure. Kidney Int; 69:184–189.

54

13.Axelrod D.M., Anglemyer A.T., Sherman-Levine S.F. Zhu A., Grimm P.C., Roth S.J., Sutherland S.M.(2014). Initial Experience Using Aminophylline to Improve Renal Dysfunction in the Pediatric Cardiovascular ICU. Pediatr Crit Care Med;15:21–27.

14.Badin J, Boulain T, Ehrmann S, Skarzynski M, Bretagnol A, Buret J, Benzekri-Lefevre D, Mercier E, Runge I, Garot D, Mathonnet A, Dequin PF, Perrotin D. (2011). Relation between mean arterial pressure and renal function in the early phase of shock: A prospective, explorative cohort study. Crit Care; 15:R135.

15.Bailey D., Phan V., Litalien C., Ducruet T., Mérouani A., Lacroix, J.; Gauvin, F. (2007). Risk factors of acute renal failure in critically ill children: A prospective descriptive epidemiological study. Pediatr Crit Care Med; 8:29–35.

16.Bagshaw S.M., Bennett M., Haase M., Haase-Fielitz A., Egi M., Morimatsu H., D'amico G., Goldsmith D., Devarajan P., Bellomo R. Plasma and urine neutrophil gelatinase-associated lipocalin in septic versus non-septic acute kidney injury in critical illness. (2010). Intensive Care Med; 36:452–461.

17.Bailly V., Zhang Z., Meier W., Cate R., Sanicola M., Bonventre J.V. Shedding of kidney injury molecule-1, a putative adhesion protein involved in renal regeneration. (2002). J Biol Chem; 277:39739–39748.

18.Bakr A.F. (2005). Prophylactic theophylline to prevent renal dysfunction in newborns exposed to perinatal asphyxia: a study in a developing country. Pediatr Nephrol; 20 (9):1249-1252.

19.Barletta J.F., Barletta G.M., Brophy P.D., Maxvold N.J., Hackbarth R.M., Bunchman T.E. (2006). Medication errors and patient complications with continuous renal replacement therapy. Pediatr Nephrol 21:842–845

20.Barnes G.E., Laine G.A., Giam P.Y., Smith E.E., Granger H.J. (1985). Cardiovascular responses to elevation of intra-abdominal hydrostatic pressure. Am J Physiol; 248:R208-R213.

21.Barrantes F., Tian J., Vazquez R., Amoateng-Adjepong, Y., Manthous, C.A. (2008). Acute kidney injury criteria predict outcomes of critically ill patients. Crit Care Med; 36:1397–1403.

22. Basile D.P., Friedrich J.L., Spahic J., Knipe N., Mang H., Leonard E.C., Changizi-Ashtiyani S., Bacallao R.L., Molitoris B.A., Sutton T.A. (2010). Impaired endothelial proliferation and mesenchymal transition contribute to vascular rarefaction following acute kidney injury. Am J Physiol Renal Physiol.; 300:F721–F733.

23.Basu R.K., Zapitelly M., Brunner L., Yu W., Wong H.R., Chawla L.S., Wheeler D.S., Goldstein S.L. (2014). Derivation and validation of the renal angina index to improve the prediction of acute kidney injury in children. Kidney International; 85:659-667.

24.Basu R.K., Wang Y., Wong H.R., Chawla L.S., Wheeler D.S., Goldstein S.L. (2014). Incorporation of biomarkers with the enal angina index for prediction of severe AKI in critically ill children. Clin J Am Soc Nephrol; 9(4):654-662.

25.Bell M., Jackson E., Mi Z., McCombs J., Carcillo J. (1998). Low-dose theophylline increases urine output in diuretic-dependent critically ill children. Intensive CareMed; 24:1099-1105.

26.Bellomo R., Auriemma S., Fabbri A., D'Onofrio A., Katz N., McCullough P. A., Ricci Z., Shaw A., Ronco C. (2008). The pathophysiology of cardiac surgery-associated acute kidney injury (CSA-AKI). Int J Artif Organs; 31:166–178.

27.Bellomo R., Chapman M., Finfer S., Hickling K., Myburgh J. (2000). Low-dose dopamine in patients with early renal dysfunction: A placebo-controlled randomised trial. Australian and New Zealand Intensive Care Society (ANZICS) Clinical Trials Group. Lancet; 356:2139–2143.

28.Bellomo R., Kellum J.A., Ronco C. (2007). Defining and classifying acute renal failure: From advocacy to consensus and validation of the RIFLE criteria. Intensive Care Med; 33:409 –413.

29.Bellomo R., Ronco C., Kellum J.A. Mehta R.L, Palevsky P.; Acute Dialysis Quality Initiative workgroup (2004). Acute Dialysis Quality Initiative workgroup. Acute renal failure—definition, outcome measures, animal models, fluid therapy and information technology needs: Crit Care; 8:R204–R212.

30.Bellomo R., Wan L., Langenberg C., May C. (2008). Septic acute kidney injury: New concepts. Nephron Exp Nephrol; 109:e95–e100.

31.Bennett M., Dent C.L., Ma Q., Dastrala S., Grenier F., Workman R., Syed H., Ali S., Barasch J., Devarajan P. (2008). Urine NGAL predicts severity of acute kidney injury after cardiac surgery: a prospective study. Clin J Am Soc Nephrol; 3:665–673.

32.Benoehr P., Krueth P., Bokemeyer C., Grenz A., Osswald H., Hartmann J.T. (2005). Nephro- protection by theophylline in patients with cisplatin chemotherapy a randomized, single-blinded, placebo-controlled trial. J Am Soc Nephrol; 16(2):452-458.

33.Berg A., Norberg A., Martling C.R., Gamrin L., Rooyackers O., Wernerman J. (2007). Glutamine kinetics during intravenous glutamine supplementation in ICU patients on continuous renal replacement therapy. Intens Care Med; 33(4): 660-666.

34.Bijker J.B., van Klei W.A., Vergouwe Y., Eleveld D.J., van Wolfswinkel L., Moons K.G., Kalkman C.J. (2009). Intraoperative hypotension and 1-year mortality after noncardiac surgery. Anesthesiology;111(6):1217-1226.

35.Boldt J., Brenner T., Lehmann A., Suttner S.W., Kumle B., Isgro F. (2003). Is kidney function altered by the duration of cardiopulmonary bypass? Ann Thorac Surg; 75:906–912.

36.Bonventre J.V. (2009). Kidney injury molecule-1 (KIM-1): a urinary biomarker and much more. Nephrol Dial Transplant; 24:3265–3268

37.Borregaard N., Sehested M., Nielsen B.S., Sengeløv H., Kjeldsen L. (1995). Biosynthesis of granule proteins in normal human bone marrow cells. Gelatinase is a marker of terminal neutrophil differentiation. Blood; 85:812–817.

38.Bourgoin A, Leone M, Delmas A, Garnier F, Albanese J, Martin C. (2005). Increasing mean arterial pressure in patients with septic shock: effects on oxygen variables and renal function. Crit Care Med; 33:780-786.

39.Bloomfield G.L., Blocher C.R., Fakhry I.F., Sica D.A., Sugerman H.J. (1997). Elevated intra-abdominal pressure increases plasma renin activity and aldosterone levels. J Trauma; 42:997-1004.

40.Brater D.C. (1981). Resistance to diuretics: emphasis on a pharmacological perspective. Drugs; 22:477–94.

41.Brophy P.D., Mottes T.A., Kudelka T.L., McBryde K.D., Gardner J.J., Maxvold N.J., Bunchman T.E. (2001). AN-69 membrane reactions are pH-dependent and preventable. Am J Kidney Dis; 38:173–178

42.Brophy P.D., Somers M.J., Baum M.A., Symons J.M., McAfee N., Fortenberry J.D., Rogers K., Barnett J., Blowey D., Baker C., Bunchman T.E., Goldstein S.L. (2005). Multi-centre evaluation of anticoagulation in patients receiving continuous renal replacement. Nephrol Dial Transplant; 20(7):1416-1421.

43.Bunchman T.E., McBryde K.D., Mottes T.E., Gardner J.J., Maxvold N.J., Brophy P.D. (2001). Pediatric acute renal failure: outcome by modality and disease. Pediatr Nephrol; 16:1067–1071.

44.Bunchman T.E. (2008). Treatment of acute kidney injury in children: From conservative management to renal replacement therapy. Nat Clin Pract Nephrol; 4:510–514.

45.Btaiche I.F., Mohammad R.A., Alaniz C., Mueller B.A. (2008).Amino Acid requirements in critically ill patients with acute kidney injury treated with continuous renal replacement therapy. Pharmacotherapy; 28(5):600-613.

46.Dai B., Liu Y., Fu L., Li Y., Zhang J., Mei C. (2012). Effect of theophylline on prevention of contrast-induced acute kidney injury: a meta-analysis of randomized controlled trials. Am J Kidney Dis; 60(3):360-370.

47.Deruddre S, Cheisson G, Mazoit JX, Vicaut E, Benhamou D, Duranteau J. (2007). Renal arterial resistance in septic shock: effects of increasing mean arterial pressure with norepinephrine on the renal resistive index assessed with Doppler ultrasonography. Intensive Care Med; 33:1557-1562.

48.Dunser MW, Ruokonen E, Pettila V, Ulmer H, Torgersen C, Schmittinger CA, Jakob S, Takala J: Association of arterial blood pressure and vasopressor load with septic shock mortality: a post hoc analysis of a multicenter trial. Crit Care, 13:R181.

49.Cameron M.A., Peri U., Rogers T.E., Moe O.W. (2004). Minimal change disease with acute renal failure: A case against the nephrosarca hypothesis. Nephrol Dial Transplant; 19:2642–2646.

50.Cano N.J., Aparicio M., Brunori G., Carrero J.J., Cianciaruso B., Fiaccadori E., Lindholm B., Teplan V., Fouque D., Guarnieri G. (2009). ESPEN Guidelines on Parenteral Nutrition: Parenteral nutrition in adult renal failure. Clinical Nutrition ; 28:401–414.

51.Cattarelli D., Spandrio M., Gasparoni A., Bottino R., Offer C., Chirico G. (2006). A randomised, double blind, placebo controlled trial of the effect of theophylline in prevention of vasomotor nephropathy in very preterm neonates with respiratory distress syndrome. Arch Dis Child Fetal Neonatal Ed; 91:F80–84.

52.Chertow G.M., Burdick E., Honour M., Bonventre J.V., Bates D.W. (2005). Acute kidney injury, mortality, length of stay, and costs in hospitalized patients. J Am Soc Nephrol; 16:3365–3370.

53.Coca S.G., Singanamala S., Parikh C.R. (2012). Chronic kidney disease after acute kidney injury: a systematic review and meta-analysis. Kidney Int; 81(5):442–448.

54.Cooper D.S., Claes S.G., Goldstein S.G. Menon, S.; Bennett, M., Ma, Q., Krawczeski, C.D. (2014). Novel urinary biomarkers remain elevated years after acute kidney injury following surgery in children. Pediatr Crit Care Med; 15:(Suppl.) Abstract No 25.

58

55.Croda-Todd M.T., Soto-Montano X.J., Hernández-Cancino P.A., Juárez-Aguilar E. (2007). Adult cystatin C reference intervals determined by nephelometric immunoassay. Clinical Biochemistry; 40:1084–1087.

56.Cruz D.N., de Cal M., Garzotto F., Perazella M.A., Lentini P., Corradi V., Piccinni P., Ronco C. (2010). Plasma neutrophil gelatinase associated lipocalin is an early biomarker for acute kidneyinjury in an adult ICU population. Intensive Care Med; 36:444–451.

57.Coulthard M.G., Crosier J., Griffiths C., Smith J., Drinnan M., Whitaker M., Beckwith R., Matthews J.N.S., Flecknell P., Lambert H.J. (2014) Haemodialysing babies weighing <8 kg with the Newcastle infant dialysis and ultrafiltration system (Nidus); comparison with peritoneal and conventional haemodialysis. Pediatr Nephrol; 29:1873–1881.

58.de Geus H.R., Bakker J., Lesaffre E.M., le Noble J.L. (2011). Neutrophil gelatinase associated lipocalin at ICU admission predicts for acute kidneyinjury in adult patients. Am J Respir Crit Care Med; 183:907–914.

59.De laet, Malbrain M., Jadoul J., Rogiers P., Sugrue M. (2007). Renal implications of increased intra-abdominal pressure: Are the kidneys the canary for abdominal hypertension? Acta Clin Belg Suppl; 1:119-130.

60.De Mendona A., Vincent J.L., Suter P..Moreno M., Dearden N.M., Antonelli M., Takala J., Sprung C., Cantraine F. (2000). Acute renal failure in the ICU: Risk factors and outcome evaluated by the SOFA score. Intensive Care Med; 6:915–921.

61.de Oliveira C.F., de Oliveira D.S.F., Gottschald A.F.C., Moura J.D.G. Costa G.A., Ventura A.C., Fernandes J.C., Vaz F.A.C., Carcillo J.A., Rivers E.P., Troster E.J.. (2008). ACCM/PALS haemodynamic support guidelines for paediatric septic shock: an outcomes comparison with and without monitoring central venous oxygen saturation. Intensive Care Med; 34:1065–1075.

62.Dent C.L., Ma Q., Dastrala S., Bennett M., Mitsnefes M.M., Barasch J., Devarajan P. (2007). Plasma neutrophil gelatinase-associated lipocalin predicts acute kidney injury, morbidity and mortality after pediatric cardiac surgery: a prospective uncontrolled cohort study. Crit Care; 11:R127.

63.Dharnidharka V.R., Kwon C., Stevens G. (2002). Serum cystatin C is superior to serum creatinine as a marker of kidney function: a metaanalysis. Am J Kidney Dis; 40: 221–226.

64.Dobrowolski L., Sadowski J. (2005). Furosemide-induced renal medullary hypoperfusion in the rat: role of tissue tonicity, prostaglandins and angiotensin II. J Physiol; 1;567(Pt 2):613-620.

65.Druml W., Fischer M., Sertl S., Schneeweiss B., Lenz K., Widhalm K. (1992;). Fat elimination in acute renal failure: long chain versus medium-chain trygliceride. Am J Clin Nutr; 5:468–472.

66.Druml W. Nutritionalmanagement of acute renal failure. (2001). Am J Kidney Dis; 37(Suppl.1):S89–S94.

67.Dussol B., Morange S., Loundoun A., Auquier P., Berland Y. (20060. A randomized trial of saline hydration to prevent contrast nephropathy in chronic renal failure patients. Nephrol Dial Transplant; 21:2120-2126.

68.Duzova A., Bakkaloglu A., Kalyoncu M., Poyrazoglu H., Delibas A., Ozkaya O., Peru H., Alpay H., Soylemezoglu O., Gur-Guven A., Bak M., Bircan Z., Cengiz N., Akil I., Ozcakar B., Uncu N., Karabay-Bayazit A., Sonmez F. (2010); Turkish Society for Pediatric Nephrology Acute Kidney Injury Study Group. Etiology and outcome of acute kidney injury in children. Pediatr Nephrol; 25:1453–1461.

69.Eades S.K., Christensen M.L. (1998). The clinical pharmacology of loop diuretics in the pediatric patient. Pediatr Nephrol;1998:603–616.

70.Edelstein C.L., Hoke T.S., Somerset H., Fang W., Klein C.L., Dinarello C.A., Faubel S. (2007). Proximal tubules from caspase-1-deficient mice are protected against hypoxia induced membrane injury. Nephrology Dialysis Transplantation; 22:1052–1061.

71.Endre Z.H., Pickering J.W., Walker R.J., Devarajan P., Edelstein C.L., Bonventre J.V., Frampton C.M., Bennett M.R., Ma Q., Sabbisetti V.S., Vaidya V.S., Walcher A.M., Shaw G.M., Henderson S.J., Nejat M., Schollum J.B., George P.M. (2011). Improved performance of urinary biomarkers of acute kidney injury in the critically ill by stratification for injury duration and baseline renal function Kidney Int; 79:1119–1130.

72.El-Husseini A.A., Foda M.A., Shokeir A.A., Shehab El-Din, A.B., Sobh, M.A., Ghoneim, M.A .(2005). Determinants of graft survival in pediatric and adolescent live donor kidney transplant recipients: A single center experience. Pediatr Transplant; 9:763–769.

73.Evans R.G., Correia A.G., Weekes S.R., Madden A.C. (2000). Responses of regional kidney perfusion to vasoconstrictors in anaesthetized rabbits: dependence on agent and renal artery. Clin Exp Pharmacol Physiol; 27:1007-1012.

74.Faisy C., Guerot E., Diehl J.L., Labrousse J., Fagon J.Y. (2003). Assessment of resting energy expenditure in mechanically ventilated patients. Am J Clin Nutr; 78:241–249.

75.Feinstein E.I., Kopple J.D., Silberman H., Massry S.G.. (1983). Total parenteral nutrition with high or low nitrogen intakes in patients with acute renal failure. Kidney Int Suppl; 16:S319–S323.

76.Felker M.G., Lee K.L., Bull D.A., Redfield M.M., Stevenson LW, Goldsmith S.R., LeWinter, M.M., Deswal A., Rouleau J.L., Ofili E.O., Anstrom K.J., Hernandez A.F., McNulty S.E., Velazquez E.J., Kfoury A.G., Chen H.H., Givertz M.M., Semigran M.J., Bart B.A., Mascette A.M., Braunwald E., O'Connor C.M. (2011), for the NHLBI Heart Failure Clinical Research Network. Diuretic strategies in patients with acute decompensated heart failure. N Engl J Med; 364:797–805.

77.Fiaccadori E., Maggiore U., Clima B., Melfa L., Rotelli C., Borghetti A. (2001). Incidence, risk factors, and prognosis of gastrointestinal hemorrhage complicating acute renal failure. Kidney Int; 59:1510–1519.

78.Fiaccadori E., Maggiore U., Giacosa R., Rotelli C., Picetti E., Sagripanti S., Melfa L., Meschi T., Borghi L., Cabassi A. Enteral nutrition in patients with acute renal failure. Kidney Int; 65:999– 1008.

79.Finfer S., Bellomo R., Boyce N., French J., Myburgh J., Norton R., SAFE Study Investigators (2004). A comparison of albumin and saline for fluid resuscitation in the Intensive care unit. N Engl J Med; 350:2247-2256.

80.Fleming F., Bohn D., Edwards H., Cox P., Geary D., McCrindle B.W., Williams W.G. (1995). Renal replacement therapy after repair of congenital heart disease in children: a comparison and peritoneal dialysis. J Thorac Cardiovasc Surg; 109:322–331.

81.Flynn J.T. (2002). Choice of dialysis modality for management of pediatric acute renal failure. Pediatr Nephrol; 17:61–69.

82.Flores F.X., Brophy P.D., Symons J.M., Flores F.X., Brophy P.D., Jordan M. Symons J.M., Fortenberry J.D., Chua A.N., Steven R.A., Mahan J.D., Bunchman T.E., Blowey D., Michael J.G., Somers, M.B., Hackbarth R., Chand D., McBryde K., Benfield M., Goldstein S.L. (2008). Continuous renal replacement therapy (CRRT) after stem cell transplantation. A report from the prospective pediatric CRRT Registry Group. Pediatr Nephrol; 23:625–630.

83.Foland J.A, Fortenberry J.D, Warshaw B.L., Pettignano R., Merritt R.K., Heard M.L., Rogers K., Reid C., Tanner A.J., Easley K.A. (2004). Fluid overload before continuous hemofiltration and survival in critically ill children: A retrospective analysis. Crit Care Med; 32:1771–1776.

84.Hartog C.S., Skupin H., Natanson C., Sun J., Reinhart K. (2012). Systematic analysis of hydroxyethyl starch (HES) reviews: proliferation of low-quality reviews overwhelms the results of well-performed meta-analyses. Intensive Care Med; 38:1258-1271.

85.Gallego N., Perez-Caballero C, Gallego A. Estepaa R., Liañoa F., Ortuñoa J. (2001). Prognosis of patients with acute renal failure without cardiopathy. Arch Dis Child; 84: 258-260.

86.Gattas DJ, Dan A, Myburgh J, Billot L, Lo S, Finfer S. (2013). Fluid resuscitation with 6% hydroxyethyl starch (130/0.4 and 130/0.42) in acutely ill patients: systematic review of effects on mortality and treatment with renal replacement therapy. Intensive Care Med; 39:558-568.

87.Garg A.X., Suri R.S., Barrowman N., Rehman F., Matsell D., Rosas-Arellano M.P., Salvadori M., Haynes R.B., Clark W.F. (2003). Long-term renal prognosis of diarrhea-associated hemolytic uremic syndrome: a systematic review, meta-analysis, and meta-regression. JAMA; 290:1360–1370.

88.Go A.S., Parikh C.R., Ikizler T.A., Coca S., Siew E.D., Chinchilli V.M., Hsu C.Y., Garg A.X., Zappitelli M., Liu K.D., Reeves W.B., Ghahramani N., Devarajan P., Faulkner G.B., Tan T.C., Kimmel P.L., Eggers P., Stokes J.B. (2010); Assessment Serial Evaluation, and Subsequent Sequelae of Acute Kidney Injury Study Investigators. The assessment, serial evaluation, and subsequent sequelae of acute kidney injury (ASSESS-AKI) study: design and methods. BMC Nephrol; 27(11):22.

89.Gillespie R.S., Seidel K., Symons J.M. (2004). Effect of fluid overload and dose of replacement fluid on survival in hemofiltration. Pediatr Nephrol; 19:1394–1399.

90.Goetz D.H., Holmes M.A., Borregaard N., Bluhm M.E., Raymond K.N., Strong R.K. (2002). The neutrophil lipocalin NGAL is a bacteriostatic agent that interferes with siderophore-mediated iron acquisition. Mol Cell; 10:1033–1043.

91.Goldstein S.L, Chawla L.S. (2010). Renal angina. Clin J Am SocNephrol 5:943–949.

92.Goldstein S.L, Currier H., Graf C., Cosio C.C., Brewer E.D., Sachdeva R. (2001). Outcome in children receiving continuous veno-venous hemofiltration. Pediatrics; 107: 1309–1312.

93.Goldstein S.L., Somers M.J., Baum M.A. Symons J.M., Brophy P.D., Blowey D, Bunchman T.E., Baker C., Mottes T., McAfee N., Barnett J., Morrison G., Rogers K.,

Fortenberry J.D. (2005). Pediatric patients with multi-organ dysfunction syndrome receiving continuous renal replacement therapy. Kidney Int; 67:653–658.

94.Golej J., Kitzmueller E., Hermon M., Boigner H., Burda G., Trittenwein G. (2002). Low-volume peritoneal dialysis in 116 neonatal and paediatric critical care patients. Eur J Pediatr; 161:385–389.

95.Haase M., Bellomo R., Devarajan P. ,Schlattmann P., Haase-Fielitz A.; NGAL Meta-analysis Investigator Group. (2009). Accuracy of neutrophil gelatinase-associated lipocalin (NGAL) in diagnosis and prognosis in acute kidney injury: A systematic review and meta-analysis. Am J Kidney Dis; 54:1012–1024.

96.Haase-Fielitz A., Bellomo R., Devarajan P., Story D., Matalanis G., Dragun D., Haase M. (2009). Novel and conventional serum biomarkers predicting acute kidney injury in adult cardiac surgery—a prospective cohort study. Crit Care Med; 37:553–560.

97.Hager B., Betschart M., Krapf R. (1996). Effect of postoperative intravenous loop diuretic on renal function after major surgery. Schweiz Med Wochenschr;126:666-673.

98.Han F., Xiao W., Xu Y., Wu J., Wang Q., Wang H., Zhang M., Chen J.(2008). The significance of bold MRI in differentiation between renal transplant rejection and acute tubular necrosis. Nephrol Dial Transplant; 23:2666–2672.

99.Hanson S.J., Berens R.J., Havens P.L., Kim M.K., Hoffman G.M. (2009). Effect of volume resuscitation on regional perfusion in dehydrated pediatric patients as measured by two-site near-infrared spectroscopy. Pediatr Emerg Care; 25:150–153.

100.Harman P., Kron I., McLachlan H.D., Freedlender A.E., Nolan S.P. (1982). Elevated intra-abdominal pressure and renal function. Ann Surg; 196:594–597.

101.Herget-Rosenthal S., Marggraf G., Hüsing J., Göring F., Pietruck F., Janssen O., Philipp T., Kribben A. (2004). Early detection of acute renal failure by serum cystatin C. Kidney Int; 66:1115–1122.

102.Herget-Rosenthal S., van Wijk J.A., Bröcker-Preuss M., Bökenkamp A. (2007). Increased urinary cystatin C reflects structural and functional renal tubular impairment independent of glomerular filtration rate. Clin Biochem; 40(13-14):946-951.

103.Herrler T., Tischer A., Meyer A., Feiler S., Guba M., Nowak S., Rentsch M., Bartenstein P., Hacker M., Jauch K.W. (2010). The intrinsic renal compartment syndrome: New perspectives in kidney transplantation. Transplantation; 89:40–46.

104.Ho J., Lucy M., Krokhin O., Hayglass K., Pascoe E., Darroch G., Rush D., Nickerson P., Rigatto C., Reslerova M. (2009). Mass spectrometry-based proteomic analysis of urine in acute kidney injury following cardiopulmonary bypass: a nested case-control study. Am J Kidney Dis; 53:584–595.

105.Ho K.M., Power B.M. (2010). Benefits and risks of furosemide in acute kidney injury. Anaesthesia; 65, 283–293.

106.Hui-Stickle S., Brewer E.D., Goldstein S.L. (2005). Pediatric ARF epidemiology at a tertiary care center from 1999 to 2001. Am J Kidney Dis; 45:96-101.

107.Ichimura T., Bonventre J.V., Bailly V., Wei H., Hession C.A., Cate R.L., Sanicola M. (1998). Kidney injury molecule-1 (KIM-1), a putative epithelial cell adhesion molecule containing a novel immunoglobulin domain, is up-regulated in renal cells after injury. J Biol Chem; 273:4135–4142.

108.Ivanišević I., Peco-Antić A., Vuličević I., Hercog D., Milovanović V., Kotur-Stevuljević J., Stefanović A., Kocev N. (2013). L-FABP can be an early marker of acute kidney injury in children. Pediatr Nephrol; 28(6):963-969.

109.Jenik A.G., Ceriani Cernadas J.M., Gorenstein A., Ramirez J.A., Vain N., Armadans M., Ferraris J.R..(2000). A randomized, double blind, placebo controlled trial of the effects of prophylactic theophylline on renal function in term neonates with perinatal asphyxia. Pediatrics; 105:849–853.

110.Jessup M., Abraham W.T., Casey D.E., Feldman A.M., Francis G.S., Ganiats T.G., Konstam M.A., Mancini D.M., Rahko P.S., Silver M.A., Stevenson L.W., Yancy C.W. (2009) 2009 focused update: ACCF/AHA Guidelines for the Diagnosis and Management of Heart Failure in Adults: a report of the American College of Cardiology Foundation/American Heart Association Task Force on Practice Guidelines: developed in collaboration with the International Society for Heart and Lung Transplantation. Circulation; 119:1977–2016.

111.Joannidis M., Druml W., Forni L.G., Groeneveld A.B., Honore P., Oudemans-van Straaten H.M., Ronco C., Schetz M.R., Woittiez A.J. (2010). Prevention of acute kidney injury and protection of renal function in the intensive care unit. Expert opinion of the Working Group for Nephrology, ESICM. Intensive Care Med; 36:392-411.

112.Jones D.R, Lee H.T. (2008). Perioperative renal protection. Best Pract Res ClinAnaesthesiol; 22:193–208.

113.Just A. (2007). Mechanisms of renal blood flow autoregulation: Dynamics and contributions. Am J Physiol Regul Integr Comp Physiol; 292:R1–R17.

114.Kainuma M., Yamada M., Miyake T. (1996). Continuous urine oxygen tension monitoring in patients undergoing cardiac surgery. J Cardiothorac Vasc Anesth; 10:603–608.

115.Kavaz A., Ozçakar Z.B., Kendirli T., Oztürk B.B., Ekim M., Yalçinkaya F. (2012). Acute kidney injury in a paediatric intensive care unit: comparison of the pRIFLE and AKIN criteria. Acta Paediatr; 101(3):e126–e129.

116.Keller C.R., Odden M.C., Fried L.F., Newman A.B., Angleman S., Green C.A., Cummings S.R., Harris T.B., Shlipak M.G. (2007). Kidney function and markers of inflammation in elderly persons without chronic kidney disease: the health, aging, and body composition. Kidney Int; 71(3):239-244.

117.Kellum JA, M Decker J. (2001). Use of dopamine in acute renal failure: a meta-analysis. Crit Care Med.; 29:1526–1531.

118.Kellum J.A., Angus D.C. (2002). Patients are dying of acute renal failure. Crit Care Med; 30:2156–2157.

119.Kellum J.A., Lameire N. (2013). KDIGO AKI. Guideline Work Group. Diagnosis, evaluation, and management of acute kidney injury: a KDIGO summary (Part 1). Crit Care; 17:204.

120.Kellum J.A., Pinsky M.R. (2002). Use of vasopressor agents in critically ill patients. Curr Opin Crit Care; 8:236–241.

121.Kelly A.M., Dwamena B., Cronin P., Bernstein S.J., Carlos R.C. (2008). Meta-analysis: effectiveness of drugs for preventing contrast induced nephropathy. Ann Intern Med; 148:284-294.

122.Kheterpal S., Tremper K.K., Heung M., Rosenberg A.L., Englesbe M., Shanks A.M., Campbell D.A. Jr. (2009). Development and validation of an acute kidney injury risk index for patients undergoing general surgery: Results from a national data set. Anesthesiology; 110:505–515.

123.Kist-van Holthe J.E., Van Zwet J.M., Brand R., van Weel M.H., Bredius R.G., van Oostayen J.A., Vossen J.M., van der Heijden B.J. (2002). Prospective study of renal insufficiency after bone marrow transplantation. Pediatr Nephrol 17:1032–1037.

124.Klinge J.(2001). Intermittent administration of furosemide or continuous infusion in critically ill infants and children: does it make a difference? Intensive Care Med; 27:623–624.

125.Koyner J.L., Bennett M.R., Worcester E.M., Ma Q., Raman J., Jeevanandam V., Kasza K.E., O'Connor M.F., Konczal D.J., Trevino S., Devarajan P., Murray P.T. (2008).

Urinary cystatin C as an early biomarker of acute kidney injury following adult cardiothoracic surgery. Kidney Int; 74:1059–1069.

126.Koyner J.L., Vaidya V.S., Bennett M.R., Ma Q., Worcester E., Akhter S.A ., Raman J., Jeevanandam V., O'Connor M.F., Devarajan P., Bonventre J.V., Murray P.T. (2010). Urinary biomarkers in the clinical prognosis and early detection of acute kidney injury. Clin J Am Soc Nephrol; 5:2154–2165.

127.Kreymann K.G., Berger M.M., Deutz N.E., Hiesmayr M., Jolliet P., Kazandjiev G., Nitenberg G., van den Berghe G., Wernerman J., Ebner C., Hartl W., Heymann C., Spies C. (2006). DGEM (German Society for Nutritional Medicine), ESPEN Guidelines on Enteral Nutrition: Intensive care. Clin Nutr; 25:210–212.

128.Langenberg C., Bellomo R., May C. Wan L., Egi M., Morgera S. (2005). Renal blood flow in sepsis. Crit Care; 9:R363–R374.

129.Lassnigg A., Donner E., Grubhofer G., Presterl E., Druml W., Hiesmayr M. (2000). Lack of renoprotective effects of dopamine and furosemide during cardiac surgery. J Am Soc Nephrol; 11:97-104.

130.LeDoux D., Astiz M.E., Carpati C.M., Rackow E.C. (2000). Effects of perfusion pressure on tissue perfusion in septic shock. Crit Care Med; 28:2729-2732.

131.Legrand M., Mik E.G., Johannes T., Payen D., Ince C. (2008). Renal hypoxia and dysoxia after reperfusion of the ischemic kidney. Mol Med; 14:502–516.

132.Le Roith D., Bark H., Nyska M., Glick S.M. The effect of abdominal pressure on plasma antidiuretic hormone levels in the dog. J Surg Res 1982, 32:65-69.

133.Levy E.M., Viscoli C.M., Horwitz R.I. (1996). The effect of acute renal failure on mortality. A cohort analysis. JAMA; 275:1489 –1494.

134.Li L., Lai E.Y., Huang Y., Eisner C., Mizel D., Wilcox C.S, Schnermann J. (2012). Renal afferent arteriolar and tubuloglomerular feedback reactivity in mice with conditional dele- tions of adenosine1receptors. Am J Physiol Renal Physiol; 303:F1166–1175.

135.Liang X.L., Liu S.X., Chen Y.H., Yan L.J., Li H., Xuan H.J., Liang Y.Z., Shi W. (2010). Combination of urinary kidney injury molecule-1 and interleukin-18 as early biomarker for the diagnosis and progressive assessment of acute kidney injury following cardiopulmonary bypass surgery: a prospective nested case-control study. Biomarkers; 15:332–339.

136.Liangos O., Tighiouart H., Perianayagam M.C., Kolyada A., Han W.K., Wald R., Bonventre J.V., Jaber B.L. (2009). Comparative analysis of urinary biomarkers for early detection of acute kidney injury following cardiopulmonary bypass. Biomarkers; 14: 423–431.

137.Lowenstein J., Schacht R.G., Baldwin D.S. (1981). Renal failure in minimal change nephrotic syndrome. Am J Med; 70:227–233.

138.Luciani G.B., Nichani S., Chang A.C., Wells W.J., Newth C.J., Starnes V.A. (1997). Continuous versus intermittent furosemide infusion in critically ill infants after open heart operations. Ann Thorac Surg; 64:1133–1139.

139.Ludens J.H., Hook J.B., Brody M.J., Williamson H.E. (1968). Enhancement of renal blood flow by furosemide. J Pharmacol Exp Ther; 163:456-460.

140.Lynch B.A., Gal P., Ransom J.L., Carlos R.Q., Dimaguila M.A., Smith M.S., Wimmer J.E. Jr, Imm M.D. ((2008). Low- dose aminophylline for the treatment of neonatal non-oliguric renalfailure– case series and review of the literature. J Pediatr Pharmacol Ther; 13:80–87.

141.Macedo E., Malhotra R., Bouchard J., Wynn S.K.,Mehta R.L. Oliguria is an early predictor of higher mortality in critically ill patients. Kidney Int 80:760–767.

142.Macias W.L., Alaka K.J., Murphy M.H., Miller M.E., Clark W.R., Mueller B.A. (1996). Impact of the nutritional regimen on protein catabolism and nitrogen balance in patients with acute renal failure. J Parenter Enteral Nutr; 20(1):56-62.

143.Manetti L., Pardini E., Genovesi M., Campomori A., Grasso L., Morselli L.L., Lupi I., Pellegrini G., Bartalena L., Bogazzi F., Martino E. (2005). Thyroid function differently affects serum cystatin C and creatinine concentrations. J Endocrinol Invest; 28:346–349.

144.Martin S., Danziger L.H. (1994). Continuous infusion of loop diuretics: pharmacodynamics concepts and clinical applications. Clin Trends Pharm Pract.; 8:10–13.

145.Mårtensson J., Bell M., Oldner A., Xu S., Venge P., Martling C.R. (2010). Neutrophil gelatinase associated lipocalin in adult septic patients with and without acute kidney injury. Intensive Care Med; 36:1333–1340.

146.Matsui K., Kamijo-Ikemori A., Hara M., Sugaya T., Kodama T., Fujitani S., Taira Y., Yasuda T., Kimura K. (2011). Clinical significance of tubular and podocyte biomarkers in acute kidney injury. Clin Exp Nephrol; 15:220–225.

147.Maxvold N.J., Smoyer W.E., Custer J.R., Bunchman T.E. (2000). Amino acid loss and nitrogen balance in critically ill children with acute renal failure: a prospective comparison between classic hemofiltration and hemofiltration with dialysis. Crit Care Med; 28:1161–1165.

148.Maitland K., Pamba A., English M., Peshu N., Marsh K., Newton C., Levin
M.(2005). Randomized trial of volume expansion with albumin or saline in children with
severe malaria: preliminary evidence of albumin benefit. Clin Infect Dis; 40:538–545.

149.Malbrain M.L., Chiumello D., Pelosi P., Bihari D., Innes R, Ranieri V.M., Del Turco
M., Wilmer A., Brienza N., Malcangi V., Cohen J., Japiassu A., De Keulenaer B.L,.
Daelemans R., Jacquet L., Laterre P.F., Frank G., de Souza P., Cesana B., Gattinoni
L.(2005). Incidence and prognosis of intraabdominal hypertension in a mixed population
of critically ill patients: a multiple-center epidemiological study. Crit Care Med; 33:315–
322.

150.Mammen C., Al Abbas A., Skippen P., Nadel H., Levine D., Collet J.P., Matsell D.G.
(20120. Long-term risk of CKD in children surviving episodes of acute kidney injury in
the intensive care unit: a prospective cohort study. Am J Kidney Dis; 59(4):523–530.

151.McBryde K.D., Bunchman T.E., Kudelka T.L., Pasko D.A., Brophy P.D. (2005)
Hyperosmolar solutions in continuous renal replacement therapy for hyperosmolar acute
renal failure: a preliminary report. Pediatr Crit Care Med; 6:220–225.

152.McClave S.A., Martindale R.G., Vanek V.W., McCarthy M., Roberts P., Taylor B.,
Ochoa J.B., Napolitano L., Cresci G. (2009). Guidelines for the Provision and Assessment
of Nutrition Support Therapy in the Adult Critically Ill Patient: Society of Critical Care
Medicine (SCCM) and American Society for Parenteral and Enteral Nutrition
(A.S.P.E.N.) J Parenter Enteral Nutr; 33(3):277-316.

153.McDermid R.C., Raghunathan K., Romanovsky A., Shaw A.D., Bagshaw S.M.
(2014). Controversies in fluid therapy: Type, dose and toxicity. World J Crit Care Med;
3(1):24-33.

154.McIlroy D.R.,Wagener G., Lee H.T. (2010). Neutrophil gelatinase-associated
lipocalin and acute kidney injury after cardiac surgery: the effect of baseline renal
function on diagnostic performance. Clin J Am Soc Nephrol; 5:211–219.

155.Metzger J., Kirsch T., Schiffer E., Ulger P., Mentes E., Brand K., Weissinger E.M.,
Haubitz M., Mischak H., Herget-Rosenthal S. (2010). Urinary excretion of twenty
peptides forms an early and accurate diagnostic pattern of acute kidney injury. Kidney Int;
78:1252–1262.

156.Mehta R.L., Kellum J.A., Shah S.V., Molitoris B.A., Ronco C., Warnock D.G., Levin
A.; Acute Kidney Injury Network. (2007). Acute Kidney Injury Network. Acute Kidney
Injury Network: report of an initiative to improve outcomes in acute kidney injury. Crit
Care; 11:R31.

68

157.Metnitz G.H., Fischer M., Bartens C., Steltzer H., Lang T., Druml W. (2000). Impact of acute renal failure on antioxidant status in multiple organ failure. Acta Anaesthesiol Scand; 44:236–240.

158.Metnitz P.G., Krenn C.G., Steltzer H., Lang T., Ploder J., Lenz K., Le Gall J.R., Druml W. (2002). Effect of acute renal failure requiring renal replacement therapy on outcome in critically ill patients. Crit Care Med 30:2051–2058.

159.Mishra J., Dent C., Tarabishi R., Mitsnefes M.M., Ma Q., Kelly C., Ruff S.M., Zahedi K., Shao M., Bean J., Mori K., Barasch J., Devarajan P. (2005). Neutrophil gelatinase-associated lipocalin (NGAL) as a biomarker for acute renal injury after cardiac surgery. Lancet; 365:1231–1238.

160.Mishra J., Mori K., Ma Q., Kelly C., Yang J., Mitsnefes M., Barasch J., Devarajan P. (2004). Amelioration of ischemic acute renal injury by neutrophil gelatinase-associated lipocalin. J Am Soc Nephrol; 15:3073–3082.

161.Moat N.E., Shore D.F., Evans T.W. (1993). Organ dysfunction and cardiopulmonary bypass: The role of complement and complement regulatory proteins. Eur J Cardiothorac Surg; 7:563–573.

162.Mohmand H, Goldfarb S. (2011). Renal dysfunction associated with intra-abdominal hypertension and the abdominal compartment syndrome. J Am Soc Nephrol; 22:615–621.

163.Moreau R., Lebrec D. (2008) .Acute kidney injury: new concepts. Hepatorenal syndrome: the role of vasopressors. Nephron Physiol; 109:73–79.

164.Mouser J.F., Hak E.B., Kuhl D.A., Dickerson R.N., Gaber L.W., Hak L.J. (1997). Recovery from ischemic acute renal failure is improved with enteral compared with parenteral nutrition. Crit Care Med; 25:1748–1754.

165.Mori K., Lee H.T., Rapoport D., Drexler I.R., Foster K., Yang J., Schmidt-Ott K.M., Chen X., Li J.Y., Weiss S., Mishra J., Cheema F.H., Markowitz G., Suganami T., Sawai K., Mukoyama M., Kunis C., D'Agati V., Devarajan P, Barasch J. (2005). Endocytic delivery of lipocalinsiderophore- iron complex rescues the kidney from ischemia-reperfusion injury. J Clin Invest; 115:610–621.

166.Myburgh J, Cooper DJ, Finfer S, Bellomo R, Norton R,Bishop N, Kai Lo S, Vallance S. (2007). Saline or albumin for fluid resuscitation in patients with traumatic brain injury. N Engl J Med; 357:874-884.

167.Nakamura A.T., Btaiche I.F., Pasko D.A., Jain J.C., Mueller B.A. (2004). In vitro clearance of trace elements via continuous venovenous hemofiltration. J Ren Nutr; 14:214–219.

168.Naftiu O.O., Vopel-Levis T., Morris M., Voeppel-Lewis T., Morris M., Chimbra W.T., Malvyia S., Reynolds P. Tremper K.K. (2009). How do pediatric anesthesiologists define intraoperative hypotension? Pediatric Anesthesia; 19:1048–1053.

169.Nejat M., Hill J.V., Pickering J.W., Edelstein C.L., Devarajan P., Endre Z.H. (2012). Albuminuria increases cystatin C excretion: implications for urinary biomarkers. Nephrol Dial Transplant; 27 Suppl 3:iii 96-103.

170.Nejat M., Pickering J.W., Walker R.J., Westhuyzen J., Shaw G.M., Frampton C.M., Endre Z.H. (2010). Urinary cystatin C is diagnostic of acute kidney injury and sepsis, and predicts mortality in the intensive care unit. Crit Care; 14:R85

171.Nejat M., Pickering J.W., Walker R.J., Endre Z.H. (2010). Rapid detection of acute kidney injury by plasma cystatin C in the intensive care unit. Nephrol Dial Transplant; 25:3283–3289.

172.Ng G.Y., Baker E.H., Farrer K F. (2005). Aminophylline as an adjunct diuretic for neonates–a case series. Pediatr Nephrol; 20:220–222.

173.Nishiyama A., Majid D.S., Walker M.III, Miyatake A., Navar L.G. (2001). Renal interstitial ATP responses to changes in arterial pressure during alterations in tubuloglomerular feedback activity. Hypertension; 37:753–759.

174.Okura T., Jotoku M., Irita J., Enomoto D., Nagao T., Desilva V.R., Yamane S., Pei Z., Kojima S., Hamano Y., Mashiba S., Kurata M., Miyoshi K., Higaki J. (2010). Association between cystatin C and inflammation in patients with essential hypertension. Clin Exp Nephrol; 14:584–588.

175.Olowu W.A., Adefehinti O. (2012). Aminophylline improves urine flow rates but not survival in childhood oliguric/anuric acute kidney injury. Arab J Nephrol Transplant; 5:35–39.

176.Orellana P., Juarez-Congelosi M., Goldstein S.L. (2005). Intradialytic parenteral nutrition treatment and biochemical marker assessment for malnutrition in adolescent maintenance hemodialysis. J Ren Nutr; 15(3):312-317.

177.Oyama Y., Takeda T., Hama H., Tanuma A., Iino N., Sato K., Kaseda R., Ma M., Yamamoto T., Fujii H., Kazama J.J., Odani S., Terada Y., Mizuta K., Gejyo F., Saito A. (2005). Evidence for megalinmediated proximal tubular uptake of L-FABP, a carrier of potentially nephrotoxic molecules. Lab Invest; 85:522–531.

178.Parikh C.R, Abraham E., Ancukiewicz M., Edelstein C.L. (2005). Urine IL-18 is an early diagnostic marker for acute kidney injury and predicts mortality in the intensive care unit. J Am Soc Nephrol; 16:3046–3052.

179.Parikh C.R., Edelstein C.L., Devarajan P., Cantley L. (2007). Biomarkers of acute kidney injury: Early diagnosis, pathogenesis, and recovery. J Investig Med; 55:333–340.

180.Parikh C.R., Thiessen-Philbrook H., Garg A.X., Kadiyala D., Shlipak M.G., Koyner J.L., Edelstein C.L., Devarajan P., Patel U.D., Zappitelli M., Krawczeski C.D., Passik C.S., Coca S.G.; TRIBE-AKI Consortium., Performance of Kidney Injury Molecule-1 and Liver Fatty Acid-Binding Protein and Combined Biomarkers of AKI after Cardiac Surgery for the TRIBE-AKI Consortium (2013). Clin J Am Soc Nephrol;8(7):1079-1088.

181.Parikh C.R., Lu J.C., Coca S.G., Devarajan P. (2010). Tubular proteinuria in acute kidney injury: A critical evaluation of current status and future promise. Ann Clin Biochem; 47:301–312.

182.Patzer L. Nephrotoxicity as a cause of acute kidney injury in children. (2008). Pediatr Nephrol; 23:2159–2173.

183.Pediatric Advanced Life Support (2000). Circulation; 102:291-342.

184.Pedersen K.R., Hjortdal V.E., Christensen S., Pedersen J., Hjortholm K., Larsen S.H., Povlsen J.V.(2008). Clinical outcome in children with acute renal failure treated with peritoneal dialysis after surgery for congenital heart disease. Kidney Int Suppl; S81–86.

185.Picca S., Dionisi-Vici C., Abeni D., Pastore A., Rizzo C., Orzalesi M., Sabetta G., Rizzoni G., Bartuli A. (2001) Extracorporeal dialysis in neonatal hyperammonemia: modalities and prognostic indicators. Pediatr Nephrol 16:862–867.

186.Plotz F.B., Bouma A.B., van Wijk J.A., Kneyber M.C. J., Bökenkamp A. (2008). Pediatric acute kidney injury in the ICU: an independent evaluation of pRIFLE criteria. Intensive Care Med 34:1713–1717.

187.Polito C., Papale M.R., La Manna A.L. (1998). Long term prognosis of acute renal failure in the full term newborn. Clin Pediatr (Phila) 37:381–386.

188.Price J.F., Goldstein S.L.(2009). Cardiorenal syndrome in children with heart failure. Curr Heart Fail Rep; 6:191–198.

189.Prowle J.R., Westerman M., Bellomo R. (2010). Urinary hepcidin: an inverse biomarker of acute kidney injury after cardiopulmonary bypass? Curr Opin Crit Care; 16:540–544.

190.Redfors B., Bragadottir G., Sellgren J., Swärd K., Ricksten S-E. (2011). Effects of norepinephrine on renal perfusion, filtration and oxygenation in vasodilatory shock and acute kidney injury. Intens Care Med; 37:60- 67.

191.Ricci Z., Cruz D.N., Ronco C. (2011). Classification and staging of acute kidney injury: beyond the RIFLE and AKIN criteria Nature Reviews Nephrology; 7:201-208.

192.Ricci Z., Iacoella C., Cogo P. (2011). Fluid management in critically ill pediatric patients with congenital heart disease. Minerva Pediatr; 63:399–410.

193.Ricci Z., Stazi G.V., Di Chiara L., Morelli S., Vitale V. , Giorni C., Ronco C., Picardo S.(2008). Fenoldopam in newborn patients undergoing cardiopulmonary bypass: Controlled clinical trial. Interact Cardiovasc Thorac Surg; 7:1049–1053.

194.Rodriguez M.M., Gomez A., Abitbol C., Chandar J., Montane B., Zilleruelo G. (2005). Comparative renal histomorphometry: a case study of oliogonephropathy of prematurity. Pediatr Nephrol; 20:945–949.

195.Ronco C., Bonello M., Bordoni V., Ricci Z, D'Intini V, Bellomo R, Levin NW (2004). Extracorporeal therapies in non-renal disease: treatment of sepsis and the peak concentration hypothesis. Blood Purif; 22:164–174.

196.Ronco C., Garzotto F., Brendolan A., Zanella M , Bellettato M.,Vedovato S., Chiarenza F., Ricci Z, Goldstein S.L. (2014). Continuous renal replacement therapy in neonates and small infants: development and first-in-human use of a miniaturised machine (CARPEDIEM). Lancet; 24; 383 (9931):1807-1813.

197.Royakkers A.A., Korevaar J.C., van Suijlen J.D., Hofstra L.S., Kuiper M.A., Spronk P.E., Schultz M.J., Bouman C.S. (2011). Serum and urine cystatin C are poor biomarkers for acute kidney injury and renal replacement therapy. Intensive Care Med; 37:493–501.

198.Rosner M.H., Okusa M.D. (2006). Acute kidney injury associated with cardiac surgery. Clin J Am Soc Nephrol; 1:19–32.

199.Sakr Y., Reinhart K., Vincent J.L., Sprung C.L., Moreno R., Ranieri V.M., De Backer D., Payen D. (2006). Does dopamine administration in shock influence outcome? Results of the Sepsis Occurrence inAcutely Ill Patients (SOAP) Study. Crit Care Med; 34:589–597.

200.Schwartz G.J., Muñoz A., Schneider M.F. Mak R.II., Kaskel F., Warady B.A., Furth S.L. (2009). New equations to estimate GFR in children with CKD. J Am Soc Nephrol; 20:629–637.

201.Scheinkestel C.D, Kar L., Marshall K., Bailey M., Davies A., Nyulasi I., Tuxen D.V. (2003). Prospective randomized trial to assess caloric and protein needs of critically ill, anuric, ventilated patients requiring continuous renal replacement therapy. Nutrition; 19(11-12):909-916.

202.Selewski D.T., Cornell T.T., Heung M., Troost J.P., Ehrmann B.J., Lombel R.M., Blatt N.B., Luckritz K., Hieber S., Gajarski R. (2014) .Validation of the KDIGO acute kidney injury criteria in a pediatric critical care population Intensive Care Med; 40:1481–1488.

203.Shapiro N.I., Trzeciak S., Hollander J.E., Birkhahn R., Otero R., Osborn T.M., Moretti E., Nguyen H.B., Gunnerson K.J., Milzman D., Gaieski D.F., Goyal M., Cairns C.B., Ngo L., Rivers E.P. (2009). A prospective, multicenter derivation of a biomarker panel to assess risk of organ dysfunction, shock, and death in emergency department patients with suspected sepsis. Crit Care Med; 37:96–104.

204.Schneider J., Khemani R, Grushkin C, Bart R. (2010). Serum creatinine as stratified in the RIFLE score for acute kidney injury is associated with mortality and length of stay for children in the pediatric intensive care unit. Crit Care Med; 38:933–939.

205.Siew E.D., Ikizler T.A., Gebretsadik T., Shintani A., Wickersham N., Bossert F., Peterson J.F., Parikh C.R., May A.K., Ware L.B. (2010). Elevated urinary IL-18 levels at the time of ICU admission predict adverse clinical outcomes. Clin J Am Soc Nephrol; 5:1497–1505.

206.Siew E.D., Ware L.B., Gebretsadik T., Shintani A., Moons K.G., Wickersham N., Bossert F., Ikizler T.A. (2009). Urine neutrophil gelatinase-associated lipocalin moderately predicts acute kidney injury in critically ill adults. J Am Soc Nephrol; 20:1823–1832.

207.Simmons E.M., Himmelfarb J., Sezer M.T., Chertow G.M., Mehta R.L., Paganini E.P., Soroko S., Freedman S., Becker K., Spratt D., Shyr Y., Ikizler T. (2004). Plasma cytokine levels predict mortality in patients with acute renal failure. Kidney Int; 65:1357–1365.

208.Singer P. (2007). High-dose amino acid infusion preserves diuresis and improves nitrogen balance in non-oliguric acute renal failure. Wien Klin Wochenschr; 119: 218–222.

209.Singh N.C., Kisson N., Al Mofada S., Bennett M., Bohn D.J. (1992). Comparison of continuous versus intermittent furosemide administration in postoperative pediatric cardiac patients. Crit Care Med; 20:17–21.

210.Solomon R., Werner .C, Mann D., D'Elia J., Silva P. (1994). Effects of saline, mannitol, and furosemide to prevent acute decreases in renal function induced by radiocontrast agents. N Engl J Med; 331:1416-1420.

211.Strazdins V., Watson A.F., Harvey B. (2004). Renal replacement therapy for acute renal failure in children: European guidelines. Pediatr Nephrol; 19:199–207.

212.Sutherland S.M., Zappitelli M., Alexander S.R., Chua A.N., Brophy P.D., Bunchman T.E., Hackbarth R., Somers M.J., Baum M., Symons J.M., Flores F.X., Benfield M., Askenazi D., Chand D., Fortenberry J.D., Mahan J.D., McBryde K., Blowey D., Goldstein S.L. (2010). Fluid overload and mortality in children receiving continuous renal replacement therapy: The prospective pediatric continuous renal replacement therapy registry. Am J Kidney Dis; 55:316–325.

213.Star R.A. (1998). Treatment of acute renal failure. Kidney Int; 54:1817–1831.

214.Story D.A., Ronco C., Bellomo R. (1999). Trace element and vitamin concentration and losses in critically ill patients treated with continuous venovenous hemofiltration. Crit Care Med; 27(1):220-223.

215.Symons J.M., Brophy P.D., Gregory M.J., McAfee N., Somers M.J., Bunchman T.E., Goldstein S.L.(2003). Continuous renal replacement therapy in children up to 10 kg. Am J Kidney Dis; 41:984–989.

216.Symons J.M., Chua A.N., Somers M..J, Baum M.A., Bunchman T.E., Benfield M.R., Brophy P.D., Blowey D., Fortenberry J.D., Chand D., Flores F.X., Hackbarth R., Alexander S.R., Mahan J., McBryde K.D., Goldstein S.L. (2007). Demographic characteristics of pediatric continuous renal replacement therapy: a report of the prospective pediatric continuous renal replacement therapy registry. Clin J Am Soc Nephrol; 2:732–738.

217.Tuladhar S.M., Püntmann V.O., Soni M., Punjabi P.P., Bogle R.G. (2009). Rapid detection of acute kidney injury by plasma and urinary neutrophil gelatinase-associated lipocalin after cardiopulmonary bypass. J Cardiovasc Pharmacol; 53:261–266.

218.Uchino S. Creatinine.(2010). Curr Opin Crit Care; 16:562–567.

219.Uchino S., Gordon D., Bellomo R.; Morimatsu H., Morgera S., Miet S., Ian T., Bouman C., Macedo E., Noel G.; Ashita T.; Ronco C., Kellum J.A.; Beginning and Ending Supportive Therapy for the Kidney (B.E.S.T. Kidney) Investigators (2004). Diuretics and mortality in acute renal failure. Crit Care Med;32:1669-1677.

220.Umgelter A., Reindl W., Franzen M., Lenhardt C., Huber W., Schmid R.M. (2009). Renal resistive index and renal function before and after paracentesis in patients with hepatorenal syndrome and tense ascites. Intensive Care Med; 35:152–156.

221.Vachvanichsanong P., Dissaneewate P., Lim A., McNeil E. (2006). Childhood acute renal failure: 22-year experience in a university hospital in southern Thailand. Pediatrics; 118:e786–791.

222.Vandijck D.M., Reynvoet E., Blot S.I., Vandecasteele E., Hoste E.A. (2007). Severe infection, sepsis and acute kidney injury. Acta Clin Belg Suppl; 332–336.

223.Waanders F., van Timmeren M.M., Stegeman C.A., Bakker S.J., van Goor H. (2010). Kidney injury molecule-1 in renal disease. J Pathol; 220:7–16.

224.Wagener G., Gubitosa G., Wang S., Borregaard N., Kim M., Lee H.T. (2008). Urinary neutrophil gelatinase-associated lipocalin and acute kidney injury after cardiac surgery. Am J Kidney Dis; 52:425–433.

225.Waikar S.S., Betensky R.A., Bonventre J.V. (2009). Creatinine as the gold standard for kidney injury biomarker studies? Nephrol Dial Transplant; 24:3263–3265.

226.van der Vorst M.M., Kist J.E., van der Heijden A.J., Burggraaf J. (2006). Diuretics in pediatrics: current knowledge and future prospects. Paediatr Drugs; 8:245–264.

227.van der Vorst M.M., van Heel Ruys-Dudok I., Kist-van Holthe tot Ech-ten J.E., den Hartigh J., Schoemaker R.C., Cohen A.F., Burggraaf J. (2001). Continuous intravenous furosemide in haemodynamically unstable children after cardiac surgery. Intensive Care Med; 27:711–715.

228.Venkataraman R., Kellum J. (2005). A. Acute renal failure in the critically ill. Curr Opin Anaesthesiol; 18:117-122.

229.Vlasselaers D., Milants I., Desmet L., Wouters P.J., Vanhorebeek I., van den Heuvel I., Mesotten D., Casaer M.P., Meyfroidt G., Ingels C., Muller J., Van Cromphaut S., Schetz M., Van den Berghe G. (2009). Intensive insulin therapy for patients in paediatric intensive care: A prospective, randomised controlled study. Lancet; 373:547–556.

230.Warady B.A., Bunchman T. (2000). Dialysis therapy for children with acute renal failure: survey results. Pediatr Nephrol; 15:11–13.

231.Wheeler D.S, Devarajan P., Ma Q., Harmon K., Monaco M., Cvijanovich N., Wong H.R. (2008). Serum neutrophil gelatinase-associated lipocalin (NGAL) as a marker of acute kidney injury in critically ill children with septic shock. Crit Care Med; 36:1297–1303.

232.White S.L., Perkovic V., Cass A., Chang C.L., Poulter N.R., Spector T., Haysom L., Craig J.C., Salmi I.A., Chadban S.J., Huxley R.R. (2009). Is low birth weight an antecedent of CKD in later life? A systematic review of observational studies. Am J Kidney Dis; 54:248–261.

233.Williams D.M., Sreedhar S.S., Mickell J.J., Chan J.C. (2002). Acute kidney failure: a pediatric experience over 20 years. Arch Pediatr Adolesc Med; 156:893–900.

234.Wittner M., Stefano A.D., Wangemann P. (1991). How do loop diuretics act? Drugs; 41:1–13.

235.Yamamoto T., Noiri E., Ono Y., Doi K., Negishi K., Kamijo A., Kimura K., Fujita T., Kinukawa T., Taniguchi H., Nakamura K., Goto M., Shinozaki N., Ohshima S., Sugaya T. (2007). Renal L-type fatty acid–binding protein in acute ischemic injury. J Am Soc Nephrol; 18: 2894–2902.

236.Ympa Y.P, Sakr Y., Reinhart K., Vincent J.L. (2005). Has mortality from acute renal failure decreased? A systematic review of the literature. Am J Med; 118:827–832.

237.Zager R.A. (1996). Rhabdomyolysis and myohemoglobinuric acute renal failure. Kidney Int 49:314–326.

238.Zaffanello M., Franchini M., Fanos V. (2007). Is serum cystatin-C a suitable marker of renal function in children? Ann Clin Lab Sci; 37:233–240.

239.Zappitelli M., Parikh C.R, Akcan-Arikan A.,Washburn K.K., Moffett B.S., Goldstein S.L. (2008). Ascertainment and epidemiology of acute kidney injury varies with definition interpretation. Clin J Am SocNephrol; 3:948–954.

240.Zappitelli M., Washburn K.K., Arikan A.A., Loftis L., Ma Q., Devarajan P., Parikh C.R., Goldstein S.L. (2007). Urine neutrophil gelatinase-associated lipocalin is an early marker of acute kidney injury in critically ill child: a prospective cohort study. Crit Care; 11:R84

241.Zappitelli M. (2008). Epidemiology and diagnosis of acute kidney injury. Semin Nephrol; 28:436–446.

More Books!

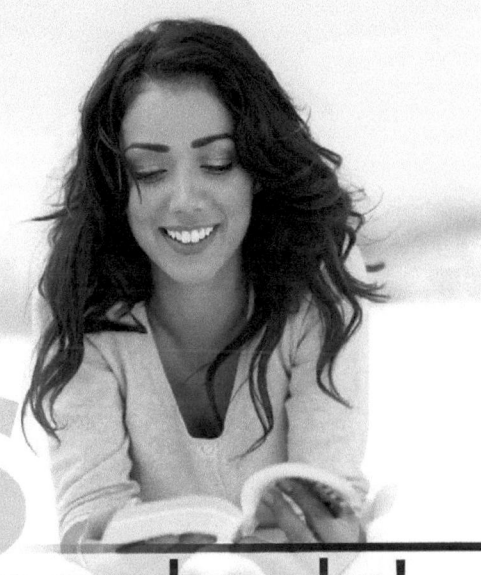

yes

I want morebooks!

Buy your books fast and straightforward online - at one of the world's fastest growing online book stores! Environmentally sound due to Print-on-Demand technologies.

Buy your books online at

www.get-morebooks.com

Kaufen Sie Ihre Bücher schnell und unkompliziert online – auf einer der am schnellsten wachsenden Buchhandelsplattformen weltweit!
Dank Print-On-Demand umwelt- und ressourcenschonend produziert.

Bücher schneller online kaufen

www.morebooks.de

OmniScriptum Marketing DEU GmbH
Heinrich-Böcking-Str. 6-8
D - 66121 Saarbrücken
Telefax: +49 681 93 81 567-9

info@omniscriptum.com
www.omniscriptum.com

OMNIScriptum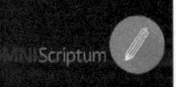

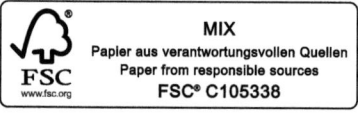

Printed by Books on Demand GmbH, Norderstedt / Germany